T0206760

Be Your Own
Medical Intuitive

Healing Your Body and Soul

Book Three in the Medical Intuitive Series

Tina M. Zion

North Carolina

Be Your Own Medical Intuitive: Healing Your Body and Soul
© 2021 by Tina M. Zion. All rights reserved.

No part of this book may be reproduced in any form or by any means, electronic, mechanical, digital, photocopying or recording, except for the inclusion in a review, without permission in writing from the publisher.

Because of the dynamic nature of the Internet, any web addresses or links contained in this book may have changed since publication and may no longer be valid. The views expressed in this work are solely those of the author and do not necessarily reflect the views of the publisher, and the publisher hereby disclaims any responsibility for them.

Limit of Liability/Disclaimer of Warranty: All effort has been done to ensure accuracy and ownership of all included information. While the publisher and author have used their best efforts in preparing this book, they make no representations or warranties with respect to the accuracy or completeness of this book and specifically disclaim any implied warranties of merchantability or fitness for a particular purpose. No warranty may be created by sales representatives or written promotional materials. The advice and strategies contained herein may not be suitable for your situation. The publisher is not engaged in rendering professional services, and you should consult a professional where appropriate. Neither the publisher nor the author shall be liable for any loss of profit or any other damages, including but not limited to special, incidental, consequential, or other damages incurred as a result of using the techniques contained in this book or any other source references.

Published by WriteLife Publishing
(an Imprint of Boutique of Quality Books Publishing Company)
www.writelife.com

Printed in the United States of America

978-1-60808-259-9 (p)
978-1-60808-260-5 (e)

Library of Congress Control Number: 2021938521

Book and cover design by Robin Krauss, www.bookformatters.com
Cover artwork by Corey Ford, www.coreyfordgallery.com
Toroidal Field illustration by Jacqueline Rogers, www.jacquelinerogers.com

Editor: Andrea Vande Vorde

Praise for
Be Your Own Medical Intuitive

"Tina Zion's expertise as a healer, teacher, and writer aligns the reader with personal empowerment—the key to any long lasting healing. She offers guidance and practical applications of scientifically and energetically based medical intuitive skills that communicate the multi-dimensional aspects of healing. This book offers opportunities for those in the medical field to maintain balance, increase their energy levels and improve their self-care so they can truly model 'wellness' for their patients. As a student of Tina's I can attest to her balanced, grounded, ethical, and thoughtful approach for maintaining connection with the spiritual worlds of healing."

—Dr. Janet Roseman,
Associate Professor, Integrative Medicine,
author of *If Joan of Arc Had Cancer: Finding Courage, Faith, and Healing from History's Most Inspirational Woman Warrior*

"Wow, just wow! Every. Single. Healer needs a copy of this book! *Be Your Own Medical Intuitive* gives Healers and Intuitives the courage, inspiration, and empowerment to look inward and bring healing to themselves. Healers spend much of their energy supporting and healing others but often feel ill-equipped to focus inward or don't have anything left for themselves after working with their clients.

Tina gently guides and reminds the healer that they are a critical link in the system and must take care of themselves first! Her book provides the tools and expertise to go inward, trust, and apply their intuition and wisdom for their own healing. After applying many of the techniques in Tina's book, I have discovered that my energy field has strengthened, I trust my intuition more and my relationship with my guides has significantly shifted. I now know that I can connect to my guides for everything and anything that relates to me. I cry tears of joy for the beautiful shifts that have occurred in my life and my own inner healing as a result of reading this book. We all deserve to heal! Thank you Tina!!!!!"

—Jennifer O'Brien
Payeur, CEO of Visionary of Nature Provides, USA

"Tina Zion works in a similar space as does Malcolm Gladwell in *Blink: The Power of Thinking Without Thinking.*

A lifetime of experience and thoughtfulness that leads one to believe that something is true, or not. Call it intuition. Can this be taught and learned? Applied to the service of health and well-being? This book provides a roadmap to just that."

—Drew Bridges, MD Psychiatrist (Retired) and author.

"Over the years I have been lucky enough to attend two of Tina's workshops. Her workshops are amazing, and Tina is a very gifted Intuitive, Teacher, and Writer.

When Tina told me she was writing a new book on how to do Medical Intuition for yourself, my first thoughts were, *How could she improve on her other two books on intuition?*

Tina's new book, *Be Your Own Medical Intuitive* has blown me away. In this book Tina's ability as an Intuitive, a Teacher, and a Writer are taken to new heights. This book takes you on a very personal journey to not only improve your intuition but also how to have intuitive insights and heal yourself. Each chapter is like having a personal mentoring session with Tina. This book was so compelling to read that I read it over a few days. At the end I could definitely feel the energetic shifts that had taken place within me. I was definitely not the same person when I finished to when I started.

It is a very powerful book that can create such amazing changes so quickly. I feel that this book is the most important book Tina has written. As she says, 'We are all works in progress' and 'to truly heal we need to heal at the energetic level.' If you want to 'truly heal,' this book is a must read. It is a masterpiece."

—Diane Reardon, Medical Intuitive & Naturopath, Australia

"Tina continues to have an unprecedented ability to translate complex physical, spiritual, and metaphysical concepts into practical applications benefitting everyone. She converts these concepts into tangible, step-by-step accessible approaches by encouraging the reader how to develop and apply intuition when dealing with varying spirits or energy forms from all realms to find and address root causes. Thanks to the depth of Tina's hands-on experience, humility, and compassion, readers, practitioners, and clients finally have a resource to not only find answers and explanations but also can execute solutions offering peace and enabling health. I can attest that I have been applying this content in my practice on a daily basis, and the consistent positive results have been extraordinary thanks to Tina."

—Maryann Kelly,
Intuitive Services Insight,
USA www.intuitiveservicesinsight.com

"Every one of Tina Zion's books is like a Bible for me and this one is no different! Her infinite wisdom paired with practical examples and simplified writing style makes this an absolute delight to read. If you are someone who wants to feel more empowered and in control of their life, then I highly recommend this book for you.

As always, I am blown away by Tina's matter-of-fact teaching for such a controversial subject. "

—Rebecca Wilson,
Medical Intuitive & Spiritual Empowerment Coach, Germany

"What an incredible book by Tina Zion! She teaches us just how powerful we are when we take charge of our thoughts and how to use that power to heal ourselves. She opens our intuition and guides us on a healing journey to not only heal our bodies but also our past, our emotions, and our relationships. She provides step-by-step instructions for each area and shows us how to find the root cause of any illness or struggle. I felt so supported and encouraged by Tina every step of the way. This book is a must have for every household because you truly can be your own medical intuitive!"

—Michelle McClintock,
Advanced Medical Intuitive,
USA www.michellemcclintock.com

"Tina's ability to examine and document her zone of genius has opened the door to a new generation of empowered healers who don't need to learn by old school trial and error. Whether you're just starting out or a seasoned veteran, you'll find her use of guides and processes powerful but yet safe. I've used them in my practice to heal many deep-rooted pains with ease and minimal time.

Be Your Own Medical Intuitive delves into areas surrounding intuition to provide clarity. It helped me examine and confirm a lot of passing thoughts I've had over the years. The processes are easy to use, provide life-changing results, and one doesn't need to be an expert to put them into practice. *Be Your Own Medical Intuitive* helped confirm a lot of passing thoughts I've noticed over the years about the mechanisms surrounding intuition. The book is easy to read, very empowering, and helped significantly improve my confidence and abilities. The knowledge I've learned from the series has been part of my daily self-care ritual, personal healing, and my professional practice.

Tina masterfully leverages a combination of carefully selected powerful words, guides, and specialists along with a collection of processes to safely and effectively heal ourselves. It is a pleasure to learn from her. *Be Your Own Medical Intuitive* is a much-needed book about self-care. There's a lot of helpful background information on why things are done a certain way, which takes away the illusion that it's not available to everyone."

—Al Danais, Canada www.aldanais.com

In Gratitude

My cherished publisher, Terri Leidich of WriteLife Publishing, frequently pointed out that the focus of my other four books was teaching practitioners how to heal others. For three years she gently told me how many people need my teachings to heal themselves. This book is because of you, Terri.

WriteLife also connected me with three other members who included me into their team. I thank Robin Krauss of Linden Design for patiently working with me to create the cover of this book. I thank Julie Bromley of Signed Books and Stuff for working together with me assisting me in so many ways, and I completely appreciate her expertise with the computer and social media. I am also delighted and grateful to work in unity with my editor, Andrea Vande Vorde. She promised me she would not alter my writing style and promised to keep my voice throughout this book, and she did just that. I also thank Cory Ford, of Cory Ford Galleries, for her unusual and expressive graphic art that has colorfully covered three of my books. I humbly declare my gratitude for each of you for being in my life and being part of my book.

I also want to declare my gratitude to every single person who reads my books, comes to my workshops, mentors with me, and takes me along in your healing journey. It is because of you that I keep moving forward, learning, growing, and writing.

"It seems we have been here only the blink of an eye by the end of our lives because it is true. Our sense of time comes from our soul memory. On some level we know this is but a fleeting moment."

—Rebecca Minser, M.D.

Contents

Part Two

Get in Charge of the Intuitive You

Part Three
Confidently Healing Yourself

Part Four

Eight Primary Causes & Your Action Steps to Heal

Appendix

Foreword

While reading Tina Zion's latest foray into the healing power of the intuitive realm, I couldn't help thinking back to my experiences growing up in Miami as a member of the silent generation. In grade school, we were taught to behave ourselves, know our place or risk being cited as "maladjusted," a judgement that would go on our "permanent record" and prelude any hope of gaining a place in society.

As it happens, during the opening day of my freshman year at the University of Miami, I came across a book by David Riesman differentiating the "outer directed" predominantly conformist personalities and the rare "inner directed" self-actualizing "free spirits." At the same time, during my first English class, the instructor claimed that everything was relative. The so-called rules were constructs designed by parents, husbands, bosses, etc. to retain power over children, wives, employees, and so forth. If that wasn't enough, David Susskind devoted his NBC talk show the following week to the primary cause of depression in America and the panel of noted psychiatrists all agreed on one single word: self-denial.

Needless to say, these revelations prompted a significant paradigm shift and eventually caused me to change my major from political science (which was relatively safe and secure in those days) to drama and first-hand encounters with an alternative universe. One that prized holding onto and then releasing the true subtext beneath characters' facades during heightened moments. A method based on the belief that those key revelations were what plays were all about so that audiences could vicariously experience all that was held in check in everyday life.

In short, I'm struck by all the exchanges Tina discloses in

her work with clients all these years later who are still deeply concerned over being weird and feel they need permission to attend to the inner and outer signals they've been receiving. As if the silent generation of yesteryear is still operative and somehow has been passed on through the decades as a sanctioned way of being. As though the primary criteria I've learned to trust over the years---the spirit of the moment---has to be validated and the gamut of intuitive self-help and self-healing needs to be carefully guided and gently released by a gifted practitioner.

Someone once wrote that the act of subscribing to what passes for normal thought and behavior only touches on, at best, ten percent of human potential. For this reason alone, Tina Zion's new book is clearly a vital antidote and necessity if we're all to lead fulfilling lives.

Shelly Frome
Professor of Dramatic Arts Emeritus
The University of Connecticut

Introducing This Book to You

"You will not find magic in your world unless you
carry magic within you."

—Robert Moss, *Sidewalk Oracles*

I want you to find your personal, private self in this book. Learn more about the intuitive you, just for you. Learn more about your intuition and energetic abilities to improve your life. Learn healing methods that have proven results. Direct healing to the exact cause of your struggles.

You may not find the exact example regarding your life, but you will find the exact origin and base of your struggles or illness. You will then find specific action steps to repair, restore, and release your struggles on all levels, in all timeframes, and in all dimensions . . . all the way to your soul.

This book is for your healing and transformation into a healthier body, healthier mind, and a cutting-edge intuitive awareness of the world around you. Allow the wisdom of your soul to shine through now.

Consider having a separate journal to record the development of your personal intuitive skills and to learn how powerful you truly are. You think you will remember everything, but as you move forward you will receive so much intuitive information that you will not recall all the important specifics. What you notice and learn about you along the way is the most precious wisdom of all.

PART ONE

Become Powerfully Intuitive
for Yourself

"You have to leave the city of your comfort and go
into the wilderness of your intuition. What you'll
discover will be wonderful. What you
will discover is yourself."

—Alan Alda

Chapter 1

What is Intuition and Medical Intuition?

"When I stopped to take a breath, I noticed I had wings."
—Jodi Livon, *The Happy Medium*

The story of your life is in your hands. The eternal story of your healing is in your hands as well.

Yes, it is harder to assess yourself, scan yourself, and heal yourself. But that is exactly what we must do. It is time for you to recognize the healer within you right now: be more in charge of all aspects of your life, create immediate healing experiences for yourself, and learn to master aspects of your life and soul. The powerful healer is really you.

We are wired to be intuitive before our birth. Even as a fetus we are receiving information regarding our biological parents, the surroundings, and the situations those parents are currently experiencing. By the time you are around six or seven years old, you have usually been taught by schoolteachers and family members that you are not perceiving what you have been perceiving. That you are just making it all up. You are naturally wired to be intuitive. You are a vital part of the entire living cosmos. Intuition is not a special gift that only a few of us have. You are intuitive too!

Intuition is purely information. People talk about trying to create balance in their lives all the time, but receiving intuitive information brings the true balance in life. True balance in life is living with awareness in the physical world and the non-physical world at the exact same time. Intuition is the most natural way to grasp, to connect, and to receive the intelligence that we humans are immersed in 24 hours a day. You have a choice to make. You truly cannot stop being intuitive, but you can certainly get in its way or simply ignore it!

This intelligent cosmos is organized, structured, and always creatively expanding. Your primary way to participate in your own personal life with awareness is to clearly receive intuitive information. It is the ability to receive information and guidance from the physical world and the non-physical world. We humans are created to receive intuitive guidance and direction. There is nothing more natural than this. You are the creator, and you can create heaven or hell or something in between.

Medical intuition is a broad, general term that constantly fluctuates between healers and energy practitioners. I teach medical intuition all around the globe and so I hear a wide range of definitions. The term "medical intuition" is about the absolute interconnectedness between our emotions, our bodies, our thoughts, our life struggles. Medical intuition is about developing a heightened level of awareness and living more in charge of all aspects of our life.

There is more to Medical Intuition than merely receiving medical information regarding the physical body, our thinking mind, and our emotions. Medical intuition assesses the impact from the environment, relationships, animals, emotions, beliefs, deceased people, alive people, traumatic events, and past lives and how they create struggles or illness for each person.

But with this information, I teach the medical intuitive to become the healer for oneself. In other words, it is not just about receiving intuitive information. It is about turning that information into a complete and permanent healing and then a beautiful, permanent release.

Allow this book to be your healing companion. Allow it to feel like I am there with you because when you utilize this book for your self-healing, I am truly there with you.

A Unique Definition

I recently realized that in my own life I identify myself as an intuitive medium but also a healer. Then my next thoughts were, "What does 'healer' or 'healing' really mean?" I quickly became perplexed. As I look back over the years of doing this level of work, I can also see that each person's outcome is often so dramatically different from one another's.

The words "heal," "healing," or "healer" seem to have become so diffused, so undefined. As I write these words at this moment, I recognize that I have been pondering the meaning of healing for a few years now. I came up with two significant ways to measure or define healing:

- Releasing of something that is a burden.

- Receiving a lasting positive effect.

When there is healing, your journey will ebb and flow, but the waves will no longer have rough highs like tidal waves do, and the lows will not plunge into the depths. The ebb and flow of life will continue like gentle ripples on a lake in the morning.

It is time for you to recognize the healer within you right now, take charge of all aspects of your life, heal yourself, and master aspects of your life and soul.

The most powerful healer has always been you.

Essential Points

- Intuition is simply the ability to notice information and attain wisdom from the physical world and the non-physical world at the same time.

- You are naturally wired to be intuitive.

- You are just as intuitive as everyone else.

- To heal is to release something and then receive something much better.

Chapter 2

Can I Really Be a Medical Intuitive for Myself?

"Our bodies communicate to us clearly and specifically,
if we are willing to listen to them."
—Shakti Gawain, Author of *Creative Visualization*

As an intuitive I've found that just giving accurate information to my clients is not enough. It seems like an oversimplification of the human sitting before me. At one point it seemed that something was dramatically missing from my time with people. So I began to include healing techniques that would end repetitive struggles or would assist in healing their thoughts, emotions, and subsequently their physical bodies.

At the end of the session, I decided to give each client homework to do for themselves. Yes, that is exactly what I did. It took me years to realize that by giving each person a homework assignment, I recognized the healer within each person. I handed the empowerment back to the client. It took my publisher, friend, and spiritual colleague, Terri Leidich of WriteLife Publishing, two years to convince me that a book was needed for everyone to recognize their own very personal healer within them.

Medical Intuition is more than just being able to scan yourself. Medical Intuition leads to a profound level of information about your eternal life's story. Medical Intuition is about identifying yourself as a soul on an amazing journey. The more you know about you, the more you are deliberately in charge of you. I love the word 'deliberately'! Can you imagine deliberately being more and more in charge of yourself and your life?

Many people tell me that they have no idea why they did what they did or why they said what they said. Do you sometimes wonder why you've blurted something out loud or done something you now regret? Are you sometimes perplexed about why you are so unhappy, so exhausted, or so ill, or why negative patterns keep repeating in your life?

You will understand why you are exhausted, ill, or finding a familiar problem constantly rising up again. You will spot more understanding, compassion, respect, and kindness for yourself. You will learn to stop fearing your surprises, emotions, fears, struggles, and your secrets because you now have multiple and specific healing methods to successfully alter the underlying energy and heal yourself.

As you deliberately take charge of yourself, you deliberately direct your future possibilities and potential, your beliefs, hidden joys, hidden pain, and not-so-hidden illness. You will know that your thoughts and emotions are living things reeling out into the universe for eternity. You will learn to take better care of yourself, and that includes the good, the bad, the ugly, and the very personal. Can you allow yourself to be who you really are meant to be? With this person's permission, here is a discussion with a client about being who you really are.

Client: When I was a child, I grew up seeing spirits and talking to spirits and getting information. But sometimes I questioned it. Am I deserving to be healed?

TZ: May I address that?

Client: Sure.

TZ: We all deserve because the aliveness in you and the aliveness in me is our spirit. So if you do not deserve it, it is like saying my spirit does not trust your spirit. It is like saying our spirit does not trust a dead person who is a spirit person without an alive body. We are all spirits experiencing life.

Client: That makes sense to me. So, my divine spirit in me deserves healing.

TZ: It is also more than deserving. We humans are a very important link in the healing system. You are a link in your own health. You can be a weak link or you can be a powerful link.

Client: I like that. This is so good. You are filling in a lot of the gaps for me. I used to stay at my grandparents' house, and I would see my other grandfather who passed away. I could see his boxer shorts and him standing in the kitchen making stuff. My mother would say that is my grandfather. I used to see my auntie and she (while in spirit) used to lay on my father when he was abusive, and he could not get up. He did not believe in this, but he could not get up. He would say, "Something is laying on me and I can't get up." There were a lot of spirits around me until I was nineteen years old when he left us. I believe now that was a lot of protection because of him. I would hear the phone ring and ask, "Why doesn't someone pick it up?" and they would say, "Because it is not ringing," and then it would ring.

It (intuition) was getting so intense that I commanded that it leave me alone. It stopped until later in my thirties it started to come back, but it is not as strong.

TZ: So you closed off your clairvoyance. If you were powerful enough to stop intuition for many years, you are powerful enough to allow it in again. Do you want to open it up again?

Client: Well, yes. I want to do this work. I have been hiding behind another profession for twenty years, but part of my sickness and my healing is that I am not being who I really am. I heard someone say you have to follow your own path to become spiritual, so now I am trying to get back to my spiritual and psychic work.

You are entering into your very own, deeply personal story. Accept everything you get . . . even the weird, and especially the weird. Weird is what unaware people tend to call everything in the intuitive world. I ask you to learn to cherish your weirdness. As you develop medical intuition, you will also become more cognizant of the natural, mystical realm of life. It is simply a matter of expanding your awareness beyond the mundane thought processes in order to receive the very subtle non-physical information around you.

You Are Already Intuitive

You already realize that you just know things about situations in your life and the lives of those around you. Some examples might be: You might already know that your heart has an energetic crack in it when you lost someone you loved. You might already be aware that every time you are with a certain family member you get a terrible headache on the right side of your head or the left side of your neck. You might be aware that the person on the phone feels "off," and the thought of fighting and arguments leap into your mind about him. You might be aware that your deceased family member comes into your dreams, especially in the last month, and you constantly think of that person but wonder why.

The following is an excerpt from a mentoring session. Notice in this session that the client already knows a great deal about his life but does not truly realize that it is intuitive knowledge, and he does not understand that the medical struggle he is having is due to the intuitive information he already knows.

Client: My integrative functional medicine physician for my gastrointestinal problem asked me why can't I do this (medical intuition) for myself? She asked me if I can work on myself, why can't I find out what is going on for myself? I told her that I do not think that is the way that spirit works. I know in mediumship it doesn't work that way. You can have your gut feelings and that kind of thing, but it is different from working with others.

TZ: Do you know why you are bringing this up right now?

Client: Well, no.

TZ: It is because I am writing my next book right now, and it is about how to do medical intuition for ourselves! Look, that is why you are bringing this up right now. It is about being intuitive for your own health and healing.

Client: Well, I have had to wait so long to get into the gastric specialist that I think I have balanced this myself.

TZ: What do you mean by "balancing it myself?"

Client: I have been working on myself without using drugs. I have worked on my own microbiome and used supplements and avoiding certain foods and now I have brought balance to my microbiome by myself. So now I know that cause of my problems.

TZ: You have been working on yourself at the physical level. You have learned the cause on a physical level but not on the energetic level.

Client: Oh, I know the cause! It was childhood . . . a very dys-functional childhood, and I was born with celiac disease. Back then there was very little help for it. My mother used to tie me up outside so I could have my diarrhea outside all day. She got so tired of it. But I have forgiven them for that. They just didn't know what to do. So, I have worked through that, and I think that has really helped rebalance this. I am asking myself to work on myself as much as I am asking my clients to work on themselves. It is very humbling. I have lived it.

TZ: Even though I have not checked in with you energetically, you have told me that you were born with celiac, and that detail should have told you something else. You came into this life with celiac . . . so you came into this life with it, but the cause came before this life. That takes us to either the cause being in a past life or when you were a fetus in your mother during this current life.

Client: I would also run away constantly, which is the other reason she would tie me up. I ran away constantly because I was convinced I was in the wrong family from the time I arrived in that family. I can see all that now as I am working with other people and that is a gift to me. I have never wanted to come back to live on this plane here on Earth and every time I come, I did not want to be here.

TZ: The more you resist it the more you will come here. You are resisting some level of awareness that you need from this Earth plane. I am asking you to adjust your thinking pattern to stop resisting coming back here to earth and embrace this level of learning here on this earth plane. You came into this life with celiac, so later after our session today, I want you to ask your guides a very clear question about the cause of you coming into this life with celiac. Ask in a very precise question to your guides. Say exactly: "Give me now the exact point of origin causing the celiac disease."

The more precise you get with your commands, the more precise your guides can get with their responses. So, to practice, ask your guides this: "Give me now the exact point of origin causing me to keep coming back to this Earth." Then see what you receive.

Client: They just showed me that I was running and hiding from them (my guides) because I am not coming back here. They are just exasperated with me.

TZ: Well, no. When they showed you that image, they were showing you that you have to keep coming back because of this resistance.

Client: Well, I will have to work on that!

TZ: Well, if you just decide right now to embrace it and get all you can get from this Earth plane, it will free you.

Client: I think that is really neat and really beautiful.

TZ: What I am trying to have you understand is that you can get this information for yourself. That is what I am trying to get across in this book. To do this level of work for yourself, you must be exactly precise with your words. If you work with your guides and you are not careful with your words, you will just get mush back. You will still be left wondering all the time about why you are not getting anywhere.

Client: Yes, we must carefully do this work for ourselves and not just for our clients.

TZ: Yes, you have to be just as careful about yourself as you are for others. When you command questions to your guides, you are not bossing around spirit. You are simply putting strong meaning and emotion to your words. That sends to them a more refined vibration so they can respond to you more clearly.

What else might you want from the guides? I will help you form a clearer question.

Client: I kept running from my guides because I did not want to come back to earth (for another life). I knew that I had so much joy here (in spirit) and I know that there is no joy on Earth.

TZ: Do you know what you just said? You have completely convinced yourself that the Earth plane has no joy. This is your greatest lesson in this life. My guides are saying that you are to create joy for yourself while you are on this Earth plane.

Client: Well, I've been working on that.

TZ: Yes, but you are convinced that it is basically a penal colony. It is up to you to create joy no matter what is going on around you on Earth.

You are already naturally intuitive. Intuitive information is in your life constantly, but most people only recognize it as strange thoughts or their wild and vivid imagination. I ask you to remember right now some of the experiences you have had that you completely put out of your mind as nothing but your brain misfiring, or your weird thoughts. It is not . . . It is your intuitive knowledge of yourself, and it is real.

Eleven Keys to Absolutely Know About Intuition

1. You are already intuitive.
2. Intuition is simply a matter of noticing in a different way.
3. Intuition will never stop feeling like your imagination . . . never.
4. You must allow yourself to receive.
5. Intuition is not a gift that only a few people have.
6. Everyone is intuitive.
7. Intuition is a learned skill.
8. Intuition is simply information.
9. Intuition is noticing the very subtle information around you and within you.
10. Intuitive information comes from both the non-physical and the physical realms.
11. You can learn the steps to intuitively learn all about yourself.

Seven Primary Blocks to Your Intuitive Skills

The blocks that I am discussing here are the primary ones that come up in all of my workshops and my private mentoring sessions. So, these are the most common struggles that I hear from people all over the world. These issues get in the way of people who yearn to do medical intuition but who struggle, in some manner, to get where they want to be. These are the primary blockages that prevent you from becoming an exceptional healer for your own life.

1. Your Worries or Outright Fears:

- **Seeing Non-Physical Beings** – I am here to tell you that deceased people are everywhere. They are at your work, in the yard, in your car, in your house, and at the stores where you shop. They are already everywhere because they are a natural part of life. We are living and breathing in the non-physical world, and it is constantly all around us and within us. You are a spirit right now, and there are spirits everywhere coming and going because they are just as alive as you are. You are a spirit among spirits. So allow yourself to perceive them. You already know they are there, don't you?

- **Being Overwhelmed** – A common question is, "What if the spirit world takes over my life?" You will notice more as you allow yourself to notice. But the most fascinating thing is that spirits will do exactly what you tell them to do. They will do what you ask because they are real people. For example, if you asked your friend to leave the room for fifteen minutes, they might think it is strange, but they would politely leave the room. It is exactly the same if you are dealing with a dead person. They will do what you say so you must take care to say exactly what you really want them to do.

- **Life Might Change** – Your life will change because you will be living a more aware and understanding life than ever before. You will understand what lies underneath other people's struggles because you have a more profound understanding of what makes you tick, and you will look out of your own eyes at the world in completely different ways.

- **Failure to Become Intuitive** – What happens if you think you have failed? Well, there really is no failure. Becoming more intuitive is about noticing the very subtle signal from the Universe. It is all about noticing or not noticing. Life is a choice between learning and then improving based on what we've learned, or stopping and not moving forward. Every split second in our lives is a choice.

- **Being Wrong** – If you are wrong in some way, then immed-iately examine how you think you are wrong. What steps did you take or not take? Learn to notice in a different way.

- **Making It All Up** – This is one of my favorite struggles to hear from someone because it is so vitally important to every single medical intuitive. Hear this now: It will never stop feeling like you made it up, imagined it, or dreamed it up. It will never stop feeling that way. Intuition is real, but it will always feel like your imagination because it is information from the non-physical realms. It is not going to be solid like we are accustomed to perceiving in the physical realm that we live in.

- **Am I Worthy to Receive Intuitive Insights?** – I was so surprised when I first heard this particular worry and con-cern. It had never occurred to me that someone would ques-tion if they were good enough. Intuition is truly only infor-mation. Granted, it is information from the non-physical life around you, but it is still only information. Do not think of it as something else.

  You are also frequently receiving information from spirit guides, angels, and even archangels. You might become aware of Jesus, Muhammad, or Buddha, or any other re-vered entity. Hear this: If they come to you, then it was their decision and not yours. That in itself tells you how worthy you are. You are in control. It is imperative that you allow yourself to receive the intuition.

- **The Spirit World Might Dominate Me** – Now this is a leg-itimate thought but does not need to be a worry or a fear. They are often confused, demanding, unaware, still feeling sick, and yes, even dead people can be afraid. Later on in this book, I will discuss the neediness of many, many deceased people. The good news is . . . they will do what you direct them to do. If you realize that you are in charge of a situation with a spirit person, there is nothing to be afraid or worried about. They are not more powerful than you are. They are really just another human in the room. If they come to you, it is because they need or want something.

- **Loving Intuitive Wisdom or the Spirit World So Much that You May Want to Leave the Physical World** – Being an intuitive and a medical intuitive is much more than interacting with dead people. The more you allow yourself to notice the non-physical world, the more you will love it. You will love it because you, as a human, are non-physical and physical at the exact same time. It brings the depth of balance that most people have been searching for throughout their lives. You will not want to leave your current life, but you will realize how alive people are even after their death. The more you receive intuition into your daily life, you will realize a richness that you have never experienced before. If life is like your cake, intuition is the luscious icing on your cake. You will feel more alive than you have ever been before.

- **What if Family or Friends Find Out I am Intuitive?** – I have noticed over many years that families are often alarmed at first when they find out you have been doing healings for yourself. People tend to judge and criticize the things they know the least about. If you do decide to share this part of your life with them then it is the exact time for you to become the teacher. Give them little bits of information at a time. I have seen this time and time again. When family and friends realize your accuracy and your healing abilities, they begin to sense the wonderment of it all and then they hold a respect for you.

- **I Have Already Experienced Strange Things and I Do Not Want That to Happen Again** – People frequently tell me that they have already had spiritual experiences that either terribly frightened them or they terribly frightened their family members. They go on to explain that they have seen inside of themselves and found something dark, or they have known about events which then actually happened in real life. They might know when someone is pregnant before the woman even knows. These are just a few examples.

My response is this: "If you do not want to be aware of those things, then what has brought you to me or to this book? Working with me will absolutely heighten your abilities." And with a surprised look on their face they often say, "Oh, I guess you are right. I guess I really want to understand what I am getting and not be afraid of these psychic things when they happen." Then I respond, "Great, that is exactly what will happen as we work together!"

- **What if I Am Not Normal Anymore?** – Living with one foot in the physical world and one foot in the non-physical world at the exact same time is the truest balance of all. You will be differently awake, knowledgeable, and mindful. You will be more powerfully aware, and this will be your new normal. Once you allow yourself to tap into the intelligence of the cosmos, you will not be the same again. You will be more.

2. Doubting or Trusting Your Abilities

"A powerful person is someone who owns their choices."
—Diane Reardon

This is a quote from a dear friend. We are on the opposite sides of the world, and yet we are connected. We trust ourselves and what we intuitively receive throughout our lives, and our personal worlds work so much better because of it.

Over and over again, people tell me that they just received intuitive information but immediately decided that the information couldn't possibly be right. Well . . . why not? Why do you think you are wrong? Why not allow yourself to be instantly correct in what you just received and how you received the intuitive information? Doubting thoughts has an energetic vibration that is thin and fragile. That weakened frequency constantly rushes through your body, diminishing your energy field. This client struggles with doubting herself.

TZ: What are the rules in your mind that you have about intuition? What is getting in your way?

Client: I really want to get intuition! In my mind I keep thinking . . . it could be this or it could be that. Then I think, what if I begin and I get nothing.

TZ: You are locked into your thinking mind. You are trying to figure things out by yourself with your logical thinking mind. You are making this moment all about your own doubtful thoughts. You are not allowing your guides to even assist you because you do not give them a chance to respond to you. What you call doubt is really you, making this all about your thinking mind and not about your spirit guides.

Client: Why am I doing that?

TZ: You are just learning and discovering one of the blocks that is getting in your way.

Trusting yourself sends a robust vibration through your energy field. The vibration of trust builds you up and sends out a vigorous signal to everyone around you, and at the same time, it sends that vigorous signal out to the universe. That in itself makes the universe recognize your signal and respond to you in a more vigorous way. Here is another revealing example from a session with this client.

Client: An old friend just kept coming up in my mind, and I just shrugged it off. Then a month later he told me he had prostate cancer. I was sensing things, but I kept shrugging it off. I should have done something about what I was getting.

TZ: Please do not beat yourself up about this. I would ask you instead to learn something about yourself and your abilities. You are very naturally picking up "something is off." So, it is a matter of learning about your process. It is about learning to trust yourself.

Client: But when I saw him a month later, I didn't get anything. Why did I get it in my thoughts a month earlier and then when I actually saw him, I didn't get anything? I know that you mention in your books that fear, doubts, second guessing ourself, and emotion will get in the way.

TZ: Well, when we are with a person that we are so delighted to see, we are not focusing on intuitive information. Emotion of delight will also get in the way.

Client: Well I have another example. I suddenly saw a black spot in this woman's right breast. I asked her if she feels any tenderness there. I mentioned it to her, and she said she is not aware of anything wrong. So that made me second guess myself and thought that I might be wrong. I have so much doubt.

TZ: We intuitives will always pick up information in the non-physical energy field that has not manifested yet in the physical. If it popped into your awareness, never doubt yourself. If intuitive information pops in, I want you to take it as an absolute truth. I never doubt it or myself. Do not diminish yourself or your abilities. You are already very accurate.

Client: When I read your book, I knew right away that my block was fear and self-doubt.

3. Do You Deserve to be Intuitive?

Intuition is a biological, inborn instinct. It has nothing to do with your actions, your lifestyle, or being deserving or not deserving. Struggling to receive the subtle intuitive world around you does not mean you are being punished. It does not signify that you do not deserve it. It only means you are not recognizing what intuition is when it comes to you. You are simply missing it when it flows to you. Thoughts and feelings of being so undeserving is a prominent roadblock for many.

Client: I constantly have that image of reaching out but feeling empty inside. I call in my sacred and divine guides who specialize in healing. I feel a difference in my heart, but I am not feeling anything else. I try a lot but never get anything. Then I thought . . . when do I talk to them? How do I talk to them? Those are my questions.

TZ: Well, first I want to ask you to back up and tell me what you are noticing about your heart.

Client: I feel I am more connected to my heart. I feel more protective of that and more like I am filling up there in my heart.

TZ: How are you doing that?

Client: I am doing heart coherence meditations, gratitude, smiling, and remembering my daughter when she was a baby. I am having closer relationships. I have been closed off and have walls up because I do not want to get hurt. People leave me, and I do not want to get hurt. I did not realize that putting walls up were actually hurting me. Letting love in is new to me.

TZ: My guides also want you to picture the most beautiful green color. They want you to imagine breathing in a bright spring green and taking it down into your lungs and then let it fills your chest and then fills your heart. Remember, energy follows human thought. You just need to think it, and it will happen.

Client: Is it also okay if I place my hands on my heart?

TZ: Absolutely, and also send the green energy from your hands into your heart.

Client: That feels beautiful . . . My heart has been craving.

TZ: What is happening and not happening with your guides?

Client: I call in the sacred and do not feel anything from it. I do not feel a physical change. I am a bit disconnected.

TZ: What pops into your mind when I ask this question: What are your expectations about the guides?

Client: Am I letting myself receive it? I am blocking them. I should feel them or sense them but I am just neutral about it.

TZ: You keep saying blocked.

Client: I think I have to do it myself!

TZ: Yes, we can do things by ourselves, but it will not be as powerful when you become the head of your team. It will be more profound.

Client: In terms of calling in extra help, I feel it is harder to call in angels. It feels like angels are much harder. With angels I am walking blindly with that. You know I connected with my guide named Maria. I sense her around me.

TZ: Ask her this, if you would. Ask her if you will be working with other guides in the future.

Client: Yes, the ascended masters. I think I need to learn more about them.

TZ: I have another thing my guides are pushing me to say to you. When I ask you this question, make sure that you take the pop as your intuitive answer from Maria. Do you feel like you are not deserving of angels and other types of divine and sacred beings to work with?

Client: I know that.

TZ: My guides keep saying the word deserving, deserving, deserving and want me to say that to you.

Client: I also have trouble with receiving and deserving. Yes, those two words. I feel like it stems from my heart. I reach out and give it all out because they deserve it and you deserve it and this one deserves it! I feel like Oprah giving cars out! You deserve it! But for me, I don't need a car. I will just walk because you can have all the cars!

TZ: Do you realize what you are saying is, the angel realm is so important and so high that you do not deserve it?

Client: Yes, but I do feel more deserving today now that I am getting some methods down. Tell me some methods in how to feel more deserving. Or is it not as simple as that?

TZ: How do you not deserve angels? Because they are too glorious? What pops into your head when I ask you that?

Client: Yes, because they are for someone else, but yes, I do deserve them.

TZ: They are waiting for you. There are all different kinds of divine and sacred guides. Do not just limit your guides to angels. They cannot learn, excel, and develop unless you allow them to work with you. Everyone is expanding and learning . . . not just we humans but also our guides. When we allow them to assist us, it affects their advancements as well.

Client: So, it is more of a collaboration and not just me taking away someone else's helper? Maybe it is just me accepting that I am deserving rather than trying to bring it in?

TZ: Exactly. Here is your next homework assignment . . . Would you ask your guide this question? Tell me or show me now the exact moment that I lost my sense of deserving.

Client: Yes, I like that.

People create all types of reasons to undermine themselves, belittle themselves, which then creates a profound struggle to be intuitive. This person created a personal rule in her mind and believed she did not deserve to be a healer for others because she was not totally healed herself.

Client: Tell me if you have ever had anyone ask you this question. I think you have probably heard everything, though. I am the archetype of the wounded healer. I am not necessarily where I want to be myself. So, I am not where I want to be. I also tell myself sometimes that I am not worthy to work with other people to heal when I have not completely healed myself.

TZ: It is not going to happen! We are never a finished product. You will never be a finished product.

Client: I feel I am not good enough and not worthy and I am not deserving until I overcome my own barriers and be on this perfect path to healing, but I never seem to get there. Why do I do that to myself?

TZ: It is because you "think" you have to be a finished product to do this level of work. But doing this level of work actually assists us in our development too. We are never going to be a finished product. Even our own guides are not finished products. The more we connect with them and work together with them as our team, the more they develop. They frequently tell me that. They say they are not finished developing either. If that is going to be your criteria, then you are always going to suffer and beat yourself up. Believe me, I am not a finished product either.

Client: I needed to hear that.

4. Your Old Rules are Getting in the Way

I am using the word "rules" to clearly explain the most powerful block getting in your way of being intuitive for yourself or for someone else. In this case, a rule is a thought that grew into a belief. That belief then became an expectation that intuition must come to you in a certain way. It must be noticed in a certain way. If you have that belief it only means that you are missing all the other ways it is coming to you.

The most dominant rule is that the intuitive must see everything with their physical eyes. If you have this rule, then everything that the universe gives to you in your mind's eye does not count as intuition, and you discard it. Seventy-five percent of what I perceive is in my mind's eye. (I will discuss the mind's eye in more depth later on.)

Many of our current rules were never really ours in the first place. When we were younger, we listened to parents or other authoritarian role models. We hear the rules they declare to us, and we tend to swallow the rules and try to believe it and apply it to our own personal life. So many times, a rule that fits for someone else is stifling in our life. You might struggle to hold on to that rule because you thought you must believe it no matter what. For example, I heard a father tell his daughter that auras are not real, and she is not seeing any colors around people. If she, as a child, decided that is a rule that must be followed, then she will struggle to see auras later as she tries to open up to her clairvoyant abilities.

Don Miguel Ruiz, author of *The Four Agreements*, states the following: "We need a great deal of courage to challenge our own beliefs." What rules do we have about intuition? Your rules become your beliefs. A belief is only a thought that you frequently have. Where did they come from? Are they positive guidelines for you, or do they stifle and restrict your awareness to receive intuitive information?

5. Your Expectations About Intuition

Oh, expectations! How dramatically interfering they are for your success as an intuitive! When I ask you this question, I want you to notice whatever jumps into your mind. What do you think intuition will be when it happens? Notice what you have already decided intuitive information is. If you have already decided what intuition should look like or show up as or how it should be, then your preconceived ideas will force you to miss all the other pathways that are coming to you.

6. I am Afraid to See Things!

Visualizing the non-physical world around you is so vitally important that we find ourselves in one of two groups. We either think that seeing is so important that we must see everything, or it is not intuition and it is not correct. The second group contains everyone else who is terrified to see anything of the non-physical world around us.

If you find yourself in either one of these groups, Group 1) Seeing is the only way to receive intuition, or Group 2) Seeing is too frightening, then you are obstructing your natural abilities.

The non-physical creation is there, and you are within it and interacting with it right now. You are a spirit, so you might as well allow yourself to perceive it visually because you are already sensing or feeling it around you anyway. A person in spirit is much less threatening than a person could be to you in the physical. A person in spirit also will do exactly what you demand that they do. (I will discuss this in more detail later in this book.)

7. What Will Everyone Think of Me?

I now teach medical intuition full time in one-on-one mentoring sessions and also a three-day workshop. During a moment of quiet, one woman asked a really good question. She hesitantly said, "What do you do with all the skeptics around you who do not believe in this stuff?" She went on, "I keep my abilities hidden because they are so critical." My response, "I simply do not give a rip in the slightest about what they think! And because I do not care at all, I never draw those people to me." There were a few seconds of silence . . . then everyone laughed and laughed.

I love this quote from Martha Graham: "There is a vitality, a life force, an energy, a quickening that is translated through you into action, and because there is only one of you in all of time, this expression is unique. And if you block it, it will never exist through any other medium, and it will be lost. It is your business to keep it yours clearly and directly, to keep the channel open."

Remember moments of feeling proud. How did that emotion feel inside of you? Remember the moments of feeling proud about someone in your life. What is the exact feeling when pride waves through you? Now . . . can you imagine feeling proud of yourself in that same way and to that same degree.

My hope for you is to experience waves of genuine pride of your intuitive development and your increasing abilities. My hope for you is to experience a deep level of comfort and security for your own health and your own perceptions. Does it really matter if some acquaintance, friend, or even a family member does not believe in your life and your life experiences? Does it really matter that you are mindful and responsive to the non-physical, otherworldly realms that exist within and around you? You are expanding your perceptions and understandings of yourself and each individual around you. You have stretched and magnified your senses, and there is still so much more to do. Can you un-expand your thoughts, your senses, and go back into a confinement so that others might be more comfortable being around you? This is only one out of an uncountable number of choices you have every single day of your life.

Stop Now and Notice Yourself with Fascination

What has been blocking your intuitive skills? In what ways do you know yourself more clearly now?

Essential Points

- Beware: We humans excel at convincing ourselves we are intuitive failures and have no powers at all.
- Look for your fears and worries. Do not try to avoid them or you cannot learn about yourself.
- Trusting yourself opens the pathway up into a wide-open highway.
- You are wired to be intuitive. You are meant to receive information through intuition.
- Deserving to be intuitive has nothing to do with your natural wiring.
- Catch yourself having subtle rules that are limiting. If you have

expectations of how intuition should be or how it comes to you, it only means that you are missing all the ways it is already coming to you.

- Realize that you live within the non-physical realms. Seeing it is natural, just like looking out from your physical eyes right now.

Chapter 3

How to Recognize Intuition When You Receive it

"A friend told me I was delusional. I almost fell off my unicorn."
—The Burlap Bag

Here is the crucial key regarding intuition.

You are constantly receiving intuitive information and, yes, even wisdom. But are you noticing it constantly? Are you noticing it at all? If not, you are simply failing to understand what intuition is, where it is, when it is, and how it comes to you.

Intuitive intelligence is not sporadic. Intuitive intelligence is constant and never-ending. It comes through animals, faces or forms in the clouds, a word or name that is painted across the side of a truck, your dreams that seem different than your other dreams, birds repeatedly coming to you, a simple phrase a child says to you, a vision that you decided was your imagination, a voice out of nowhere that called your name, a meaningful moment that you decided to call a coincidence instead of a blessing, a breeze that touched your face and moved your hair just as you finished your prayer.

Imagination or Intuition?

Read this next statement. Hear its truth and take it deep into your soul: Intuition will never, ever, ever stop feeling like your imagination.

Read that over again because it is so important.

It will never stop feeling like you just imagined it because intuition is information on a vibrational level. It is coming from the non-physical universe that is within you and surrounds you at the same time. It is not solid like the chair you are sitting on. When it comes to you it will never stop feeling like you just dreamed it up or made it up in your mind. Did you really take in that information just now? It will never stop feeling like you just invented it. Once you make this leap you are on your way to becoming a skilled intuitive for yourself.

This interaction is a superb example of how powerful and constant intuitive information is coming to us for ourselves and for others. We simply do not recognize it as intuition or intuitive wisdom.

Client: I began to teach the toroidal field to one of my clients, and I got a very awkward response from her and almost a defensiveness and a resistance to doing it. It was curious and no relevance to it.

TZ: I must interrupt. It is extremely relevant. You got an intuitive hit about her, but you are blowing it off. Why are you blowing it off as not relevant?

Client: Well, when I began talking to her about the toroidal field, bringing in the energy and how it worked, I could just sense her like . . . well, no! So, I just did not take it to heart. I offered it to her so she could take it if she wanted, but she did not want it. It was an offer, and she did not want it.

TZ: You were actually receiving another level of information. You were picking up an intuitive hit about her, but you did not recognize it as intuition. You were picking up resistance from her for some reason. Now the reason for the resistance or the cause is important. Something would not let her learn to "power up" her own energy field (more on the toroidal field later).

Client: Ahh . . .

TZ: Had you recognized it as intuitive information, you could have brought up to her that you are picking up a feeling of resistance. You might have said, "I am picking up some resistance. Let's talk about it and tell me what you are noticing." You would have then looked for the cause of the resistance to become stronger, brighter, and bigger, which is what the toroidal field does for us. Resistance to power up could be coming from an interference such as by a deceased person or from an alive person or an event in her childhood.

Client: That is brilliant!

TZ: Hopefully this is a really good teaching situation, and I am thrilled that you brought it up. Something is causing resistance within her, to become beautiful and big and powerfully bright . . . What the heck? Something is blocking her.

Client: That just makes so much sense!

TZ: She has a fear or an interference causing this resistance.

Client: This is so wonderful. I need to learn to open up and be receptive about what is right in front of me. I am learning how to do that. See, I did not think twice when that happened with her.

TZ: What you did not notice is how power-packed that situation was for your client and you. You received the deeper level of information, but you blew it off and tried not to take it as an insult to you. What you received at that moment was probably the basis of all of her struggles.

Notice and Receive the Very Subtle

I mention all the time that I simply teach how to pause and notice the very subtle signals of life around you and life within you. That is the fundamental truth of it.

Pause—Slow down for only a split second. During the split second of the pause, you send your "awareness sensors" all around your own body, then send your "awareness sensors" out into the world around you. Do this for only a second but frequently.

Notice—Do not look for what you hope to find within or around you. Notice as the most fascinated observer. Notice without criticism no matter who it is. Notice only what is actually happening with interest. Now notice as if you are an eagle or an angel looking out over the more comprehensive greater picture of things.

Noticing does not mean working hard to find intuition. Noticing and searching for intuition are direct opposites of each other. We humans are literally antennas meant to receive information around us. Antennas do not put any effort into it at all. They very passively receive electrical information that comes to them. We humans are antennas. Stop working and struggling and start gently noticing. Everything that you notice around you and everything that happens around you and happens to you can be taken as important intuitive information. There are no accidents. Even accidents are not accidents. The world around you is speaking to you every second of every day. You only need to notice.

Sometimes your personal message is literally a word or an image on a billboard along the highway. I am giggling as I write this because 99.9 percent of the time it will not come to you as physical as a billboard. But . . . occasionally, it will be in a material form like that.

Receive—The wisest people in the world are the ones who notice everyday life around them. They are the ones who are fascinated with the sky, events, people, and nature and find meaning in everything. For example, I was on a phone meeting when I turned to look out the window just as a hawk swooped by, nearly touching the building with the tip of its wing. I immediately shared that with the person on the phone and he exclaimed that hawks have great meaning to him. Notice that I felt it had meaning and this man confirmed that he recognized it as an intuitive sign. That sign in that split second of a moment gave him a direction to take in his life.

Do you see how we both noticed it, then took it as intuitive information and a profound signal from nature? I had no idea that birds were important in any way for this person. And yet something made me turn to look out the window in the same split second that a hawk rushed by, and at the same time he was telling me he was trying to make a decision. I trusted that moment as a piece of information because there is meaning in everything. This man on the other end of the phone trusted it as a meaningful communication for the next segment of his life.

Everything has meaning. It is just a matter of pausing, noticing the subtle, and allowing yourself to receive the meaning.

Six Pathways to Receive Intuition

Where is intuition? How is it coming to you right now? Intuitive knowledge is all about receiving. It is only a matter of noticing the subtle. We receive the information but do not realize the pathways whereby it is coming to us. Here is a brief interaction during one of my mentoring sessions:

Client: When I looked at the arm, I saw dots on the palm, and I got the instant impression of gravel. I got a picture of gravel in my head. I also felt tightness in the wrist.

TZ: Now let's really look at these examples that you just mentioned. Let's start with tightness. How did you actually receive the signal of tightness? Because you are actually receiving energetic informational signals. So how did you actually receive "tightness"?

Client: It was more of a knowing. Like with the gravel, I saw gravel in my head and then the word "gravel" popped into my head. But with tightness, it just felt tight.

TZ: I want you to slow down and deeply realize that you just described at least three pathways from which you received medical intuitive information. You received information in thoughts, which is telepathy. You received it in a wave of knowing, and then you visually saw gravel. I want you to know that you are rocking it. You just received intuitive information through sight in your mind's eye, through waves of knowing, and also through thought. Do you hear what I am saying? Three pathways. And this time, you did not "work at it." Remember, working hard at it has been getting in your way until now.

Client: Okay, that is good. I am trying to stop working hard. I just sat there looking at it. I didn't try to pick up anything.

TZ: Exactly. We are antennas. They do not run around trying to find the information. It just sits there and waits for information to come to it. Working so hard trying to find intuition has been your only block to becoming an intuitive.

Here are the pathways to notice, receive, and then acknowledge it as informative wisdom.

1. **Your Own Body Sensations:** Your body communicates with you regarding two differently focused pathways: internal information or external information.

- **Internal Signals Within Yourself:** Your body constantly speaks to you about yourself by sending you energetic signals. The clearest example is physical pain. There is always emotional pain underneath physical pain. The location of your physical aches and pains also gives you yet another more profound level of information. To explore this more deeply I want you to sense that pain in your right foot is probably sending you different information than a pain in your heart. Here is a simple example of different meanings that your body might speak to you about. An ache in your heart that happened during meditation might signal to you that your heart center just expanded in new and positive ways due to the waves of love surging throughout your body. A pain in your right foot could signal to you that you are afraid to take the next step forward by leaving your old job to go into a new career.

- **External Signals From Other People:** Your body also signals you about other people. For example, I was sitting with a friend, and the longer I sat with him, the more delighted I felt. I noticed that the delight seemed to be coming from him to me. I finally asked him what is going on that he is feeling so delighted? He answered, "How did you know! I just learned that I got a new position at work that I wanted so much. But I am not supposed to tell anyone yet!" Externally, he did not seem any different, but I kept noticing happy energy coming toward me and an upward lift in my own body. I was receiving intuitive information in my own body about another person. I received that information by feeling an upward lifting sensation within my chest, and I kept sensing a lovely floating-like feeling. I did not sense those things until I was sitting for a short time with the other person.

I have another example that describes how we pick up signals regarding other people within our own bodies. Again, I was meeting with a new friend. When I sat down with her, I began feeling very itchy, and I sat there scratching more and more. My new friend finally asked if I had a skin condition. I said no, not at all. My friend then said, "Well, I am covered with psoriasis, so I was wondering if you are too." Do you see how I was picking up an energetic signal from the other person and it was accurate?

Your body is picking up energetic signals from those around you. I want you to realize that you are not getting someone else's conditions or illness. You are more intuitively aware of vibrational signals from other people around you. The signals from others can be their feelings about you or signals of their thoughts and emotions about their own life and physical body. This can happen when you personally know the people but also from strangers who have simply walked past you.

It is vital for your own well-being and self-knowledge to sort out what your body is telling you. In other words, your body speaks to you about yourself, but it also picks up energetic signals from anyone around you. It is all about noticing whatever you notice and to trust what you notice.

2. **Your Sense of Taste and Smell:** These senses seem to be the least recognized as a pathway for intuition to come to us. The best examples are the ones that people mention in my mentoring sessions. People tell me that they smell roses or lilacs or the smell of the ocean when their grandmother is there. Many say that their father used to smoke cigarettes while others say they smell pipe tobacco. A family member told me that she used to live in an old house and often at night the kitchen smelled like canned soup cooking on the stove. And then my friend said, "It wasn't me! I cannot stand canned soup." She felt that it was a deceased male tenant who used to live in the old house before her. This man must have eaten a lot of canned soup. She realized that even in spirit form, he was there with her, sometimes reliving a moment in time with his soup.

3. **Your Hearing:** I want to describe this pathway (clairaudience) more specifically. If we were talking on the phone right now, you would be hearing the sound of my voice as it touches your eardrum. Sometimes, we intuitives will truly receive a particular sound or a strong voice as if someone is standing next to you or talking to you on the phone. That is the intuitive pathway of hearing. In my experience, that external voice or sound happens, but not very often.

When I ask people to describe how they are hearing spirit, they begin to describe something quite different. They describe clear thoughts leaping into their heads, their brain, or their mind. That is a different pathway known as telepathy which is thought vibrations shooting back and forth between two or more individuals in the living or the non-physical realms. That is different than hearing a voice as if a person is talking to you inches away from your face.

4. **Your Thoughts (Telepathy):** I am convinced that this is the most misunderstood and ignored pathway to receive intuition. This is the primary pathway. Telepathy is the energy of thought transmitting back and forth between individuals. It is the primary way we receive information but the least recognized. What generally happens is you feel that your own thoughts are constantly getting in your way.

So, until now, you "think" that your thoughts are all your own and they are intrusive and interfering with your intuitive abilities. But now realize that thought is a prominent pathway to receive information. Your guides respond and answer you, but you think you are making it up. Also, when you talk to your deceased loved ones, they try to respond to you but most of the time you talk over them, do not take a moment to listen for your guide's answers, or you discount their answers as your imaginative mind making it all up.

Every single word we think has its own energetic vibration. A string of words in a sentence we think in our heads has its own energetic vibration. These thought frequencies are real things, and they radiate throughout your body and also flow out beyond your skin, creating a portion of your aura. Your positive or negative emotions then empower the energy of each thought.

5. **Your Knowing:** This pathway is difficult to describe, but I will try.

It is a strong current of information all blended together that contains a significant viewpoint, idea, or topic. For example, you might know that your family member is pregnant even before she knows. You might know that you are about to meet a new friend. And then that person comes up to speak to you at a meeting a week later. One more example could be that you sense a knowing that the primary colors in your own aura are pinks and purples. Yes, you can have a knowing of colors and not visually perceive them. (More about the meaning of colors later in this book).

6. **Your Seeing:** Please absorb this into your awareness now. Do

not make seeing everything more important than all the other pathways. I place it last to send a message to you that seeing intuitive information is not the most important. If you make seeing more important than the other routes, you are basically neglecting and disregarding all the intuitive information that is surging though the other pathways. If you continue to make seeing so important, you are abandoning about 80 percent of the intuitive evidence that is trying to get through to you.

Most people who are beginning to open up to their natural intuitive abilities think they will see the spirit world just like they do the physical world around them. You will rarely see the non-physical world that solid because it is not solid. You will sense the alive essence, and it is usually wavy and completely transparent.

You usually will not see your deceased loved ones as solid as they were when alive. If anything, you will see more of an impression of a male or female and the impression of their age and clothing. Non-physical beings will have some vague form but little definition. The impression will often be a hazy outline of a human, your deceased pet, a spirit guide, or a fairy-type being for example.

Stop Now and Notice Yourself with Fascination

Are you responding to the signals or ignoring them? What do you notice happens when you ignore your body signals? Illness perhaps? What does your body tell you right now as you read this? (I will discuss this in the Body, Mind, and Emotional Connection later in this book).

Where is Your Mind's Eye?

Seeing within your mind's eye is just as accurate and real as seeing with your eyes open. In fact, it will be extremely clear information because it came in through your mind's eye without a tidal wave of distractions from the physical world. The evidence will be pure and free of clutter as it enters into your mind's eye.

The energy center in your forehead (the third eye) is the primary intake center for intuition. In the center of the brain lies the pineal gland, or the seat of the mind's eye. My nursing book many decades ago had one sentence about the pineal gland. It stated that the gland is a mystery. The authors of that nursing book did not know that the pineal gland energetically functions as headquarters for our most natural intuitive abilities. It is the receiver and processor for intuition and the human.

This person thinks: Must she see everything with her physical eyes open?

TZ: Here is one of the main problems that most people have with being intuitive. They think they have to see everything with their eyes open. They think they have to see spirit guides with their eyes open. They think they have to see deceased people with their eyes open. Apparently, I am pretty good at this and probably 80 percent of what I "see" is with my eyes closed. I am seeing within my mind's eye.

Client: Yes, you are right, that is what I think I am doing. Right now, I think I cannot see my new guide as I look around, so I think I am failing.

TZ: Close your eyes. Call out to your guide now and notice whatever you notice in your mind's eye and do not work at it. Simply notice.

Stop Now and Notice Yourself with Fascination

I ask you to notice the sensations within your forehead. Does it feel like it is pushing outward or flowing inward?

An outward sensation will tell you that you are trying way too hard to find intuitive information.

An inward flow will tell you that you are gently receiving intuition without working hard to get it. This fluid reception is more natural. We humans are intake centers. We receive intuitive wisdom. We must pause and receive evidence without working and toiling away at all.

Eyes Open or Eyes Closed?

Working together, the third eye energy center and the pineal gland accomplishes the intake and processing functions. The third eye energy center also performs like an old-fashioned projector shining out to a screen to be observed, casting intuitive intelligence through images. It projects an uncountable amount of intuitive data in visual images, numbers, symbols, and tiny movies. This is why seeing with your eyes closed is as important as seeing with your eyes open. In short, the ability to see non-physical intuitive information, clairvoyance, has two pathways within it. Perceiving with your eyes open and your eyes closed.

For a long time, I assumed that everyone's mind's eye projected images to the same location that my images are projected to. I see images in my mind's eye that actually show up in the back of my eyelids. I thought everyone's mind's eye projected images onto the back of their eyelids as well . . . but I was wrong.

I was teaching a large class in New York and sharing with the students where they will find their projected images. One very brave student in this class slowly raised her hand and said, "I am seeing my mind's eye projecting in an entirely different place than you are describing."

"Really? Where is yours showing itself?" I said.

Then other people raised their hands to declare that theirs is also in many different locations too. I was amazed as the entire class and I explored each person's place where their third eye images show up.

Should I see with my eyes open, or is it okay to see within my mind's eye?

Client: Sometimes in my meditations people's faces come into my mind, and I do not even know them. They just appear in my mind. Sometimes I have seen them on the street, but most of them I have no idea who they are. Then words like "guilty" or "shame" come into my thoughts, so I know that they are in need. I see this with my eyes closed. They talk to me in my mind. Many people I do not even know.

TZ: You are already very advanced in your abilities to receive information.

Client: Yes, but I ask myself, "Why is this happening?" I ask myself, "Is it in their physical body or their emotions?" I ask myself, "What do they need?" But I do not get any information.

TZ: You just stated that you ask yourself many questions about the visions you just had. Then you say that you get nothing back. Is that correct?

Client: Yes.

TZ: Well, instead of asking yourself, I want you to ask your questions to the people that you are seeing in your mind's eye, or I want you to ask questions to your guides. I do not want you to call out to any guide floating past you. I want you to call out and ask for the most evolved ones, and the words to use to get the best are: Divine, Sacred, Pure, Holy guide. When you use those powerful words, that rules out all the rest.

Client: There are different kinds of guides then?

TZ: Yes! There are different kinds of guides, but there are also plain dead people who think they can be a guide. Some of them are deceased family members who think they can be your guide. My grandmother wants to guide me, but she has not reached the highest level of the divine and sacred. (My grandmother is still a beautiful assistant in my life but not a divine and sacred guide.)

Client: That makes sense. Sometimes I feel in my heart when a guide feels high or not high. If I feel afraid then I know it is not good. Sometimes they feel very light and happy. For example, I saw the face of a man, and it looked like Jesus, and I felt a hug. Then I thought . . . Jesus just hugged me. But I did not see who it was.

TZ: Wait a minute! You just said you saw an image of a man in your mind, so you did see. I want you to really be aware of that. You did just see the face of a man, and the thought came to you that it is Jesus. Now did you "see" with your eyes open or eyes closed?

Client: I always see with my eyes closed.

TZ: I almost always see with my eyes closed too! About 80 percent of what I see is in my mind's eye. Now this is important for you to understand. Most people I work with in mentoring sessions tell me that if they see it with their eyes closed, they do not count it at all. They think it is nothing and discount it as nothing.

Client: It is impossible for me to say it is nothing because it is so real. But why do I not see much with my eyes open?

TZ: Well, I see maybe 20 percent with my eyes open. The reason we do not see so often with our eyes open is that our eyes are so used to seeing very solid things in the world around us. Our physical eyes are not used to seeing things that are not physical such as spirit people.

When I see a person in spirit, it will not look like you see me now. It will look more like an impression or an outline of a human. They cannot hold the energy that long to be seen so physical because they are not physical.

Client: Oh, that makes sense!

I personally see intuitive information in the back of my eyelids as if the back of my eyelids is a movie screen for images, symbols, and tiny movies. Here are other examples where many people, from many classes, describe the location of their inner sight shows up:

- I am seeing the image in the center of my head.
- I am perceiving about three feet out in front of me.
- It's in my right temple area of my head.
- I see images in the back of my skull just under the bone.
- Everything shows up about six inches in front of my face.
- My location moves all over the place.
- It is all in my heart chakra.

Stop Now and Notice Yourself with Fascination

The first step is to stare at an object in the area around you right now. It does not matter at all what the object is. Memorize the object in detail. Then close your eyes and notice that the object you just studied will show up somewhere. That is your location. Now you know yourself in a new and meaningful way.

Receiving Symbols

Symbols quickly tell a story. Business cards, billboards, websites, and flags are just a few examples that blast symbolic information at us on a daily basis. Designs and logos are extremely important ways to send immediate signals to potential customers and clients. How many times have you picked up a business card and it seemed like nothing happened within you, so you tossed it without another thought? How often have you looked at a business card that appealed to you? A swift wave of energy connected you to that person or company. Business cards tell an instantaneous story through symbols.

Spirit guides frequently use symbols because it efficiently gets an entire message across to us. Everything within a symbol is a precise piece of information. To get that message clearly, you need to notice all the details within the symbol. Let's say you just asked your spirit guides a question, and the image of a box of tissues leaps into your mind's eye. Pulling tissues out of the box and crying immediately pops into your thoughts. You just received a signal that prompted a thought that led you to realize you have tears inside of you that need to be cried.

Intuition Pops Like Popcorn

This is one of the most critically important pieces of information in this book. Intuitive knowledge will always leap into your awareness like a kernel of corn exploding into a piece of popcorn. The clearest intuitive information will be instant or sudden. Focus on whatever pops into your awareness. Always take the pop! Whatever comes into your mind immediately after the pop will not be intuitive information. Everything after the immediate pop is your analytical thinking mind trying to sort out what just happened. Your thinking mind's job is to explore, investigate, and scrutinize something. It does this constantly, as it should, to help you organize yourself and the things of life. This brain process of analyzing is not intuition.

I have come to trust the information that pops for a simple reason: my analytical thinking mind did not have time to alter the information. Images, thoughts, names, or ideas that catapult into your mind from out of nowhere will always be the clearest intuitive information. Use the "popping of information" as a guidepost. Information that springs into your mind instantaneously will always be the clearest and truest intuitive information. Always trust the pop!

Dreams, Nightmares, and Night Terrors

Dreams are another pathway to receive intuitive knowledge and communication. However, we do not usually consider dreams to be a pathway for intuition. Some dreams are literally your brain trying to sort out and make sense out of the life you have been living. However, many dreams are not just dreams. They are your genuine experiences.

We humans are not dormant lumps as we sleep. We are extremely active and living our lives. Many situations, events, meetings, travel, and communication happen during our dreamtime. We travel during our sleep, which is also known as astral projecting. We interact with our loved ones who are in spirit. People who are in the living also reach out to us, or astral projecting, sometimes whether we want them to or not.

We also astral project and initiate contact with living people whether they want us to or not. We learn. We teach. We go to other dimensions. We sometimes circle the world on a mission of some type.

Personally, for example, in nearly 100 percent of my dreamtime, I meet with groups of people I do not know. I rarely know anyone in my dream state. I am in different countries with different people in different cultures. I always seem to teach or work with people in some manner. We often try to figure things out or plan new goals for the future. A mentoring client in the United Kingdom asked if she could tell me about a dream that involved the two of us together.

"I would like to share a dream I had of you last night. Before you came into the dream, I saw this bird, which was beautiful. She was all the colours of the rainbow. I couldn't get over how close she was to me. I heard the word "imminent" and then the bird left. You and I were in somewhere that looked like a castle. It was very posh. You were showing me what looked like letters that were in gold. The lettering was just below the ceiling line of this room. The letters could only be seen when you shined a light on it, then they would disappear. I'm sure that the letters looked like italic letters and I'm sure there was a message."

I frequently receive emails from people about their dreams because I am in them. Many times, they do not even know who I am, but I have popped up on their computers and then popped up in their dreams. They say I come into their dreams to help them in some way or to teach them. Here is an interesting example of another person's dream which offered validation and evidence that we humans are living an active life even while we sleep. Someone recently described her dream to me in this delightful, comical way.

"You were in my dream recently. I walked into a large room that was all golden. You were up in front of the group teaching them something serious. When I walked in you stopped talking, looked directly at me, and stated, "Do not ever be late again!" I quickly took my seat and got my books out of a bag. The very next day after I had this dream, my daughter brought some things over to my house in a bag. It was the exact same bag that was in my dreams the night before."

I am laughing again as I write this. What is also quite validating is that this person had never taken a class with me in the physical world at that time. She did not realize before this dream that I am a stickler for starting a class on time and for each person being there on time too. Here are the realities in this tiny dream example:

- I teach classes in my dreamtime constantly.
- I wake up knowing that I was teaching in a specific country.
- It really is important to me to begin a class on time.
- I actually ask people attending my courses to be on time.
- I do not wait for them if anyone is late to my class.

We humans make unquestionable connections with other living people in our dreamtime. Deceased people we knew in life actively make connections with us. If you are honest with yourself, you will notice that these dreams do not really seem like our regular dreams. This type of dream feels much more real and often emotional. People in spirit are honestly doing their best to make contact with you. Spirit people will come to us much more during our dreamtime after making many attempts to speak with us during our awake time. If deceased people frequently show up in your dreams, you probably ignore them or don't recognize them during the day.

Yes, we receive intuitive information and have intuitive non-physical experiences even during our sleep. Many times our dreams are about struggles that we currently have, or struggles that have happened in the past. Unresolved trauma can rise up in our dreams as a nightmare. One of the common symptoms of post-traumatic stress disorder (PTSD) are nightmares where we relive the event. It can also come as unrecognizable dreams that seem unrelated to the actual trauma. Our subconscious relives the event and the emotions of the event over and over because it attempts to resolve and heal the event. This may continue on for years after a trauma in our life.

I have noticed that nightmares that are thought of as night terrors seem to have a common element. Something or someone is about to attack them in some way. For example, many women and men secretly tell me that they wake up in the night with the feeling that something is crawling on top of them, trying to suffocate them, or standing over them in some way as they lie in bed. They often describe an inability to move or fight. This is commonly known as sleep paralysis. Western medicine explains this in physiological terms. I want you to also consider another cause. I ask that you also consider that it might be caused by a negative person in spirit who was an aggressive perpetrator in the life they just died from.

When people leave their body at death, they do not automatically become angelic. They leave their body simply with the awareness level that they have at their time of death or that they had within that life.

If that person lived a life consumed with being a sexual perpetrator, for example, then the weight and darkness of that energy continues to engulf the spirit of that person. They still focus on those obsessions. On a much lighter note, if the previous owner of your home was committed to and obsessed about their property, that energy continues to be their focus after death.

Most people suffering from this intrusion think it is a horrible dream or their vivid imagination. But the cause of many of these night terrors is a person in spirit. I find that working with the deceased person and assisting him to cross over stops these shocking sleep time moments. For now, please realize that even nightmares and night terror events are intuitive information happening. (Action steps to release aggressive deceased people are later in this book.)

Synchronicities: Pivotal Moments

In *Sidewalk Oracles*, the author Robert Moss states, "You will not find magic in your world unless you carry magic within you."

The term "synchronicity" is used when multiple events happen at the same time, giving that moment a deeper sense of meaning. The most pivotal moments in our lives are often synchronicity events and yet I notice that most people do two things with profound synchronistic moments: they immediately diminish it and decide it is a "meaningless nothing," or simply see it as a quirky coincidence.

Animism is the principle that everything is alive, that there is a common thread of spirit or soul in all objects in the material world such as animals, mountains, plants, rocks, water, birds. This connection interweaves throughout all things as well as all moments. It interweaves us humans into the tapestry of the alive planet that we live on. Everything has meaning because we humans hold a vital part in the "everything" of the universe. You are not separate from anything. We are part of a complex network of communication.

There is meaning in all things happening within us and all things surrounding us. Signals may come from the cosmos or from the physical realm. It might come as numbers, lyrics from a song that repeats and repeats inside your head, trying to get its message across to you. It can be a photo on a billboard or a sign in front of a church that leaps out at you when you drive past. The signals may enter your dreams or appear as words on someone's T-shirt in the checkout line of the store. It can come from a stranger who walks up to you at the bus stop and innocently says one beautiful sentence full of wisdom. That stranger had no idea that her little comment just took your breath away and at the same time answered the question in your mind.

A client gave an excellent example of synchronicity when she said, "Yesterday afternoon, I clicked on a free short webinar, and the opening line that the speaker said was: 'Stop giving yourself away!' Wow, that is exactly what you had said to me! No coincidence there!" That is living in the magic of life.

Since we live in an electronic world of computers, the Universe can more readily use electronic devices to send us signals and messages. Here is a true example.

Client: I had an experience I want to share with you. I had to reset my password for something on the Internet. It was tiny lettering, and I was being so careful. it was nearly fifty digits. I finally got to the end of the password, and it said that it was not entered correctly. It also highlighted the section that I had made the error. You will not believe this, but it said, "x ray eyes." That was not me!

TZ: Wow! What do you make of that? (My workshop is entitled: Become a Medical Intuitive: Seeing with X-Ray Eyes)

Client: I have had experiences of spirit coming through electronics before.

TZ: Do you know why?

Client: No, not really.

TZ: Because our physical body when we are alive is very electrical. Medical tests such as an EEG, EKG, and an EMG are measuring the electrical movement of the brain or the heart or the muscle. The paddles that emergency people place on someone's chest is shooting electrical surges into the heart to shock it into action. This is because each heartbeat is set off by an electrical spark of energy. The entire human body is very electrically alive.

So, it is really the spirit that is electrically alive, and that allows the spirit to more easily alter electronics such as an alarm clock, ceiling fan, or computer. I have heard from many people that their deceased loved one's name suddenly appeared on the screen and their name had never been used in those programs or that computer.

A woman in Wales emailed me to say that my photo instantly jumped onto her computer screen. She went on to say that she was not looking for an intuitive teacher, but there I was! She knew it was so strange that it must be a message for her. So, she went to my website, looked me up, and has been mentoring with me for over two years now. She has her own clients and is now known for her readings and healings.

Stop Now and Notice Yourself with Fascination

Notice the environment that you are in at this second. You may be in a commuter train with many others, you may be in a restaurant reading as you wait for your meal, you may be in a home in the country, or an apartment high up among the clouds, or on top of a picnic table in the park. Please take just a moment to receive something from the world around you. Allow yourself to receive the tiniest message from world around you.

Signals from Your Environment and Nature

I was in an action-packed day of writing this book but stopped at eleven a.m. to switch my computer to a virtual meeting program for my eleven a.m. mentoring session. My client began by stating that she was completely blocked and very afraid to open up an emotional state she had as a child. She went on to describe how her family strongly scolded her for saying insights she was naturally perceiving from the spirit world around her. She quickly learned the family rule to not talk about spirits.

As we discussed how her old rules were really her family's rules and not her own, I clearly saw Archangel Michael, in all his glory, standing behind the client in the back corner of her room. As soon as I asked her to allow herself to be aware of an angel's presence in the room, my client said she knew it was Michael and he was in the corner of the room behind her. She finally allowed herself to be aware of the high energy intuitive wisdom around her.

Now, here is the even more exciting detail about this story. The client's dog suddenly but calmly walked into the room, jumped up onto a chair, turned away from the client and away from the computer screen where I was located and stared into that same corner of the room. Now, please know that it was a bare corner without windows or any other distraction that might suddenly draw a dog's attention.

That dog had his back to us, all the while staring directly at Archangel Michael in the corner. I finally asked the client to turn around and observe what her dog was doing. When she saw that her dog was staring at Archangel Michael, she was amazed. Her dog was validating that the Archangel was truly there. My new client received a clear signal from the animal world that what she was noticing in the non-physical realms was honestly there.

A moment recently happened in my own life. I sat on my porch in a prayerful, thoughtful moment and sent a request out to the universe regarding a conflict between myself and someone else. My guides told me to send healing to the conflict and the person involved. I occasionally use a pendulum to dowse, so I dowsed with the pendulum and commanded goodwill to be placed immediately into the situation and all people involved.

My eyes were closed until I felt the energy shift toward the good and positive. I opened my eyes to see if the pendulum had stopped yet. I did not notice the pendulum because there was a glowing bright pink dove right in front of me. It looked directly at me but was so motionless that I immediately decided it could not be real. I stared at it and it stared at me. We both sat motionless. It broke the enchantment of the moment when the bird moved to pick at something on the ground. But it continued to glow a brilliant pink.

If nature delivers signals to us, what on earth was the message from a normally gray bird that radiated a brilliant pink color and staring at me? For centuries, doves have been symbolic of peace. Pink is synonymous with the vibration of unconditional love from the heart. That was my message, and from an extraordinarily eerie, surprising, and stunningly beautiful messenger. The second I grasped its meaning, the dove flew away. That is the magic of communicating with the energy of the cosmos.

A dear friend called me in a terrified panic. She turned into her driveway late in the afternoon and slammed on her brakes. All across the top peak of her house sat at least twenty vultures. These birds eat the dead. They are not killers. These birds create fear in people because it is assumed it is a sign that someone is about to die. This is exactly what rushed through my friend's mind and body.

This is why we must examine the details about an animal or bird's life to understand the exact message that it is sending to us. We must examine the way it lives, its characteristics, and how it does what it does in its life. Studying the details of nature leads you to interpret the clearest, most distinct message for our lives.

In this case, upon examination, the vulture does not kill its food. It assimilates and absorbs something that has already died or ended. It does not cause the death. Its signal is to understand and transform whatever in our lives has just ended. It is about change and releasing something in your life that recently ended and transforming it into something positive, nourishing and something that we learn from. This is a great example of how important it is to look into the details of how the bird or animal lives in order to receive the most well-defined and purest message for your life.

Just yesterday, I was in the middle of a mentoring session with a client when I looked out the window and saw a mother deer and her two fawns. At the moment the deer and her babies arrived, I mentioned it to the person I was meeting with. I asked her to receive a message from the deer and the two fawns who just arrived. She tearfully exclaimed that she was just about to tell me about her two children. One who was alive and doing well and the one who passed on in childhood.

I want to share a few other examples of nature sending signals and messages. For the most part, owl sightings are rare. Owls, however, came directly to me three or four times in my life. The rare times that owls physically came to me was in bright daylight, which is yet another level of rarity. As I drove down a road, I noticed an owl up ahead, sitting on a utility pole. I slowed down, inching along at a walker's pace. Just as I pulled up so I could see the owl through my side window it plunged to the ground, grabbed its prey, and looked up into my eyes.

Another time an owl swooped across the hood of my car as I turned into my driveway. And yet another example of owls signaling me happened as I got out of my car in a parking lot. The owl plunged out of the sky and landed on the ground in front of me, turned around, and looked me directly in the eye.

Nature constantly responds to you because you are not separate from it. You may ask a question from inside your heart and then ask for a signal. Immediately you hear a light wind rustling through the trees as it approaches from the far side of the woods. The coolness touches your face and feels like a blessing just brushed through your hair. No. It is not a coincidence. You received an answer in that moment.

A hailstorm of insects splattered my windshield so thick that I had to pull over to clear it away as best I could before I drove on. I had never experienced anything like that before. The next day I stopped at four gas stations to actually wash off all the smears on the windshield. Not any of the four stations I stopped at had windshield cleaner. I just drove quite a few miles between gas stations attempting to find some. You might ask, "What is the moral of this bug story? How can that be an intuitive message from spirit?"

The meaning of my bug trauma is simple and became quite clear to me. Many things were "bugging" me in my life at that time. To see this life situation clearly, I must stop all actions, and it will take some effort to cleanse myself of the aggravation. Once I make the effort to cleanse and heal myself the road ahead will be in clear view.

These are only common examples of how life speaks to us in tiny but monumental story moments. It is up to you to notice that a living message is happening around you and for you. Notice the details and you will see how the circumstance applies to your life. The story will also guide you toward the path to resolve it.

Signals from Numbers

Numbers are simply symbols, and just like any symbol, numbers have their own vibrational meanings and signals.

I spoke with a client who described a moment that just happened to him. He said, "I received a gift today. Six deer ran past me during a walk outside." He was thrilled by that, but then he went on to say that one of the deer stopped and walked toward him, stopping only six feet away. He even took out his phone and took a photo of the deer. Four things to notice:

1. The number six came into his life twice in this moment. Six deer and six feet near him. So, what does the message of six mean to him personally?
2. How do deer live their lives and what characteristics do they have?
3. What do deer mean to him personally?
4. He called it a gift. What does a gift personally mean to him in that moment of his life?

Another client told me that he was seeing the same numbers everywhere. He saw pairs of double-digit numbers such as 12:12, 10:10, 11:11 on his clocks, license plates on cars, people's addresses on their homes and mailboxes. I only asked him to notice the perfect balance of these figures. The message might be to live a more balanced life, or for this individual it might mean he is to notice patterns repeating in his life and that could be healed.

I sat with my aunt and uncle. My aunt randomly mentioned that Uncle Burt has been waking up every night for months at 2:22 a.m. I nearly choked on my coffee. I too had been waking up at 2:22 a.m. every night for many weeks. Then a week later one of my clients told me he was waking up every night. He continued to say that he looks at the clock each time and it is always 2:22 a.m.

When these synchronistic messages happen with music, people, nature, or some other pathway, we intuitives can offer a basic interpretation, but it is always best for each individual to note the details about their message, study the details as a symbol full of information, then apply the details to their current life.

Quickie Guideline for the Meaning of Numbers:

#1: New beginnings, leadership, taking action.

#2: Partnerships, balancing all things, harmony.

#3: Creative, unique, playful, lighthearted.

#4: Stable, dependable, secure.

#5: Experimenting, adventure, change.

#6: Empathy, understanding, unconditional love.

#7: Spiritual, intellectual, looks for hidden truths.

#8: Abundant, successful, lucky, accomplished.

#9: Closure, transformation, preparing for the new.

#11: A master number—Symbol of a gateway to higher wisdom of the universe.

#22: A master number—Partnership and balance between the physical and spiritual.

#33: A master number—To envision and to manifest love, com-passion, blessings.

Signals from People Around You

I held back tears as I stepped into the elevator. I had just left my attorney's office. He told me that I would never make more than minimum wage, and I'd better get all I can from my divorce settlement. All I heard was how, yet again, I was a failure and this distinguished authoritative person declared that my entire financial future was bleak. The elevator door opened, and a man stood in the corner. Since I was in such grief, I barely noticed him. I just entered, turned, and looked at the door, as most people do in an elevator.

Ever so softly, I heard the sounds of a canary singing. The stunning, crystal-clear sounds of a canary grew a little stronger. I looked at him and smiled. This man just looked at me so lovingly as he continued to whistle the canary music from the ninth floor down to the lobby. The door opened, so I stepped out. I turned to thank the man for lightening my soul. There was no one in the elevator, and the door closed.

One of my most cherished synchronistic moments happened when I was admitted to a hospital.

As the physician left my room, I said, "You are so great!"

He said, "I tell my kids I'm superhuman, but if I really was, I could stop your illness. He turned from me and walked toward the door. Then he said over his shoulder, "If I was superhuman, I could look into you with X-ray vision eyes." Click went the door. That emergency room physician had never met me before. He had to look at my chart to see what my name was, and yet he used the term that has been the title of my workshop for over ten years. The title of my workshop is, *Become a Medical Intuitive: Seeing with X-Ray Eyes."*

Notice the intuitive messages from the environment, nature, and people around you. Examine the features and qualities of everything about the event. Then translate those characteristics into information that the universe created just for you. Incorporate this precious intuitive information as a truth into your everyday life. The more you learn from the universe around you and within you, the more flowing and effortless your individual life becomes. You are no longer resisting or denying its absolute structured wisdom.

Signals from Déjà Vu

Robert Moss stands out as he beautifully describes déjà vu in this way.

"By my observation, the dream self is forever tracking ahead of the ordinary self, scouting challenges and opportunities that lie in the future. Its expeditions leave trace memories of the future that come alive when we enter a scene we have dreamed."

The French phrase, *déjà vu*, translates literally as "already seen." As I considered putting a déjà vu section into this book, I decided to look up the dictionary's definition which is, "The illusion of remembering scenes and events when experienced for the first time." Illusion means a false idea or a false belief.

For the first time ever, I was struck in the face as I read the definition. One of our unseen human skills and abilities are boiled down to an illusion, a false idea. Period. The end. The medical and psychological professions seem to dedicate themselves to blocking and rejecting our unseen powers because they cannot be seen. So, if it cannot be seen within the human body's physical structure, or a person's psychological behavior is outside of the norm, it is judged as an illusion, as nonexistent. If I could boil it down to one statement, I declare that this only means that the medical and psychological professions are so focused on the physical world that they have not allowed themselves to experience their own unearthly powers and abilities.

My dear friend Maggie once told me that she finally got to go on vacation to Salem, Massachusetts to see the area of the historical witch trials. She walked into one of the homes that visitors are allowed in. She immediately had a déjà vu experience. Mary saw herself in that exact corner of the house before she actually arrived there. She knew what was in the home and where it was sitting. She also spontaneously saw flashes and heard the sounds of her own past life that she had lived many centuries ago in that same location.

Time is not linear. It does not have a beginning and an end. We are much more than a body that travels through time as though there is a beginning, a middle, and an end. We humans are each a spirit, and that spirit within us has very few limitations. It is not limited like our physical body is. We can stretch backward, forward, and even stretch out to other locations. We can stretch ahead into our future potentials. We can stretch back even into our past lives. Déjà vu is re-experiencing or remembering a moment in what we call our future.

Steps to Receive Synchronistic Messages:

1.   Do not ignore or overlook the event, even if it is odd or unusual. Notice even more because it is odd.

2.   Recognize the details of what just happened as a powerful piece of information just for you.

3.   Know that you are not making it up. It is the universe signaling you.

4.   Study the details of the event such as sounds, exact words, actions, no actions.

5.   Notice the characteristics of the animals, birds, or nature.

6.   Allow these details to be a unique message just for you.

Stop Now and Notice Yourself with Fascination

Synchronicity is the world naturally communicating with you. Allow it to be a natural part of your life now.

Form a clear simple question about your life.

Send your question out to the universe with the expectation of receiving an answer.

Be on high alert for the message.

I ask you to now be a vigilant observer always on high alert! Acknowledge synchronicity as it happens to you. Be on high alert to recognize these moments of messages as the universe comes together to speak to you in symbolic stories. Each time is magical twinkling in your personal life. Examine the details of these occurrences to receive the details of your special message. The more aware you become, the more in charge you are of you and your life.

I want to take a moment to point out to you that I am not offering a synchronicity dictionary for you to look up the meaning of everything. It is up to you to grasp the symbolism of events, certain moments, conversations, the environment and nature.

It is up to you to allow the message to come to you. This is truly important to understand.

Essential Points

• Be vigilant and on high alert for repetitive signals or patterns.
• Everything has meaning.
• It is up to you to notice, receive, and apply the information for your life.
• Synchronicity is magical, but it is not magic.
• Synchronicity is the cosmos speaking to you.

PART TWO

Get in Charge of the Intuitive You

"You know—when you start getting really clear
about what you desire and want in your life it's
amazing what, when, where, and how things
start showing up."

—Tammy Barton

Chapter 4

Your Thoughts are Directing Everything

"Ideas are projected as a direct result of the force by which
they are conceived and they strike wherever the brain
sends them by a mathematical law comparable to that
which directs the firing of shells from their mortars."

—Honore de Balzac

I constantly hear statements such as these:

"I cannot help how I think."

"I cannot stop how I think."

"I was raised this way and that's all there is to it."

"I have always been negative because my mom was negative."

"My whole family is angry, so I am angry all the time."

"This is just who I am, and I can't do anything about it."

If you are not in charge of your thoughts, then who on earth is in charge of you? Who is running the show, so to speak? You think you are simply a finished product of your childhood and have no choice of who you are? Is it truly that simple? I guess it can be that simple if you want it to be. But there could be so much more for you.

If we condense life's purposes down to the general basics for every human being on the planet, we can describe it in three primary categories:

• You constantly have free will to make choices.

- You have constant opportunities to learn, to take new actions, or do the same thing all over again.

- You constantly have experiences to learn and to expand your awareness and wisdom.

I texted my dear friend that I was in a flurry of writing my new book. I joked around and asked if she had any wisdom that she would like for me to quote in my new book. There was a long silence on the other end of the phone, then we visited for a bit more, and then we hung up. A couple of hours later, my text ring went off. Here is Janie's wisdom for us:

"Life on earth is short. However, it is a long time to live in an encumbered state of confusion, emotional pain, or under religious doctrine that simply does not feel right. Those gut feelings mean something and are meant to be paid attention to. Opening oneself up to the belief that there is more to our existence than we can physically see is one of the greatest gifts you can give yourself."

Wow, Janie K. Thank you.

The mystics throughout time were mystical because they understood and knew how to use the power of thought and emotion. They understood that all things have a spirit of aliveness. They understood how to use their abilities to direct and alter the environment and people around them. You do not need to be a mystic from ancient times to carry out magical changes within you and around you.

We are powerful because we are human. Many people think humans are weak victims of life. We humans are meant to be powerful because we are a vital link in the system of the cosmos. We are not meant to be the weakest link. We are not meant to be victims of the universe. We are meant to own our empowerment and utilize it for ourselves and for each other. Feel and understand that you and I, and every human on this earth, are key figures within an intelligent system. We are key figures not only for ourselves but in the lives of others as well.

This is why the non-physical world responds so readily for us. When you call out to the non-physical realms of our guides, angels, and healing beings, they respond. They will not interfere in your life without an invitation and a clear request. It is not because we are weak. It is because you are an important link in the structure and the organization of the Universal system. You are important, not weak.

We are creators. Our brain functions as a computer. Our mind, however, is everywhere. I will repeat that. Our mind is everywhere. Your mind is electrically alive and is in each and every physical cell of your physical body. It emanates beyond your skin and is commonly known as the aura. The mind is within our soul, and it makes up our soul. Your brain is the computer and your mind is the internet with a natural access to the world within you, the material world around you, and the infinite world beyond this world.

Your energy is electrical in nature, vibrating at certain frequencies. Each and every frequency holds informational signatures within it. Everything is energy, and energy is information. The human body and brain receive and send energy. We humans are vibrating electrical forms living within an electrically vibrating world. You can be a powerful link in the electrical system, or you can be a weak link. It is totally up to you.

Think of the magnitude of that! If we can alter non-physical energy into an illness, what on earth might we be capable of doing with positive, loving thought energy? The most significant and powerful concept I will say in this book is this:

You are already creators on the most subtle yet most important level of all: energy.

For example, a client just today told me that a long time ago, she received painful intuitive information about her husband. She stated to the universe, "Stop this intuitive information forever!" Her intuition stream of information stopped immediately at that moment. It stopped because that is how powerful we are. Our relationship with the Universe and the earth that we dwell on is guided by our thoughts and emotions.

The universe shifts and changes with every change that we go through. Every change of thought, emotion, or energy alters the universal energy around you. It varies because you are an intricate part of the whole. As you shift, the universe shifts and changes and adjusts.

Everyone has stuff in life, even the ones who are considered experts. It all depends on what you do with the stuff that is yours. My hope for you is to stop feeling as if life is throwing you around and then stomping you into the ground. My hope is for you to stop feeling blindsided by someone or something. My hope for you is to be in charge of you and your experience of life.

We are so much more in charge of our lives, our experiences, and our situations than we will probably ever know. I am driven and determined to assist you, if you allow, to gain wisdom and a multilayered understanding of just how in charge you are.

What You Think, You Manifest

Science has discovered that energy follows along with each human thought. Science has also discovered that human thought strongly affects physical matter. Every person's thought energy affects the environment of this physical world we live in.

Your head is connected to your body. Your mind is the energy that vibrates throughout the body's system of cells, blood, bones, tissue, organs, and muscles. Your mind interconnects thought, emotion, and the body. Nothing is separate. One component affects all the others. What we think creates emotions, and emotions vibrate throughout the body. Positive emotions create well-being while negative emotions create disease.

Our thoughts are profoundly powerful because each one emits a vigorous energy signal to your body, to your soul, and outward to the world. Each word has its own electrical spurt. Each sentence is a string of words that combine into yet another vibration. Each vibration carries an unbelievably potent message. Those mental messages surge through your body and rush outward and into the external world around you. Science now declares that our human thoughts alter the physical world. You are more powerful than you can even imagine.

First notice what you are saying to yourself about the world around you. For example, "I cannot stand the way people treat each other. I can't tolerate the news anymore. I can't see the hardships the woman in the grocery store must be having."

Now notice what you are saying to yourself about yourself. Stop yourself, get in charge of you, and deliberately shift your thoughts and your awareness into the positive. Here are some examples:

- "I have been so grouchy lately. I am taking charge of me and turning it into happiness right now."

- "What am I learning from the difficult experience I am in right now?"

- "I am going to learn from that event that happened to me when I was a child."

- "I was born with this disability, so I am determined to learn more about me and my soul."

- "I used to drink too much, so now I am learning about emptiness in my solar plexus and filling it with my own empowerment."

You have manifested everything that you are witnessing in this moment. You have even manifested this book in the same moment that you are looking around and assessing your environment.

If you are struggling to manifest success in any way, you must lovingly examine your worthiness. Do you truly feel in your mind and heart that you deserve to receive what you yearn for? I first became aware of this particular struggle while teaching my *Become a Medical Intuitive* course. We were exploring as a group the old, old rules that have been getting in each person's way.

Each person yearned to do medical intuition for others and yet they felt blocked, blank, or confused instead. During our group exploration, someone called out, "I do not deserve to help people at this profound energetic level." The large class agreed that was the basis of their own struggles as well.

You can only manifest what you feel you deserve, and you can only manifest success when your thoughts can conceive, feel, and picture that which you yearn for.

Stop Now and Notice Yourself with Fascination

What are you manifesting now? Just take a moment to look around you right now no matter where you are or what you are doing.

Visualization

Do you know that many Olympic athletes are trained to visualize the perfect action for the sport they are performing? They are trained to visualize every muscle, each stretch, the tension, the feeling of lifting off the ground and flying through the air. They visualize themselves in amazing detail and imagine the feel of each action. When you visualize but also feel the sensations and emotions of the visualization, you send a coded, detailed message to your body and the environment. It is like studying a map first and then following it in a more effortless way. They visualize deliberately to achieve a goal.

Visualization is also one pathway to receive intuitive information. Spirit shows us a tiny movie as a way to give us an instant and valuable segment of information. Visualizing that movie is clairvoyance. The intuitive movie might seem to float in the air in front of you or it might show itself to you within your mind's eye. Both locations that your visions display themselves to you are equally important.

Are You an Analytical Thinker?

Usually half of the groups attending my workshops hold their hands up to say they are analytical thinkers. Those same people are completely convinced that their analytical mind interferes with their intuition. Your thinking mind is your strongest pathway to receive intuition.

A mentoring client described her struggle to intuitively figure out what she intuitively received. She said, "Well, first I think it might be this, and then the next moment I wonder if it might be that. I am just not getting clarity. I am not getting clear messages from my guides." As she talked, she demonstrated with her hands and arms. "You know what I mean. It is like pulling cooked spaghetti apart."

Oh my goodness, I laughed and laughed because this woman brings me such delight.

I told her I must use her spaghetti demonstration in the new book I am writing. But then I said, "Susie, you clearly described what our thinking mind does. That is not how we receive intuition through the pathway of thought. The thinking mind examines this option and then another option and then tries to figure out preferences, choices, and alternatives. That is what it is supposed to do to sort things out."

The intuitive mind, however, pauses for a split second, and receives the pop of intuitive information in the form of thoughts. It does not assess, examine, select, or measure. It receives intuitive information that does not fluctuate. Intuition remains steady about an issue or decision and does not alter. If you are trying to pull apart cooked spaghetti, you are in your analytical mind and not your intuitive mind. (More about this in the pathways to receive intuition.)

Take Great Care of Your Abilities and Your Empowerment

The greatest and most important choice you have to make in this life is to make this one decision. Will you use your powerful abilities for the greatest good for yourself and others, or will you use it to gain power over others?

Working on your self-awareness is truly the purpose of living the human life. Attempting to work on others without their direct and clear permission is completely different, extremely complicated, and highly risky. Do you see and sense the difference? As your personal strength and empowerment builds, be highly aware that you may feel the need to enlighten everyone else around you. You may want others in your life to grow exactly as you are growing. Resist the urge to drag others along your personal path. Others may not be ready.

Five Essential Warnings Against Working on Others for Your Own Healing:

1. Permission, permission, permission is essential. I cannot declare this strong enough. Never, ever attempt any energy work without receiving verbal permission or clear intuitive permission from the person you want to send energy, healing, or changes. Do not try to pull these people into the Light and do not try to change a person "for their own good." This power is real. Using your energy to push another in a direction that you think is best for them is abuse of your abilities. Permission keeps you functioning on the side of Light and Love. It keeps you from slipping into the darker side of life.

2. If you send energy without permission it means that you have decided something is wrong about another person. Your decision is based more about you than the other person. It is based on what you believe, what you want, or what you hope for.

3. Do not deceive yourself by thinking it is for their own good and send energy anyway.

4. Do not try to bend this guideline by asking the other person's higher self instead of asking the individual.

5. You could be pushing your will onto others and altering a

path that the other person is supposed to experience and potentially learn from.

Trust Yourself and Be Proud

One of the common struggles I hear from people is they do not trust themselves and they do not trust that the intuitive information they get is correct. Trust is complicated. It is a vital part of excelling as an intuitive for your own well-being.

Each thought is an electrical burst of energy. Trusting or not trusting are simply two thoughts that create two different beliefs, and those beliefs create two different emotions. If you do not trust something, then you create a narrow, jagged vibration that rushes from you and out into the world. That irregular vibration hinders the physical world and non-physical world's response to you. It will also draw distrustful people to you.

The thought, belief, and subsequent emotion of trusting self and the non-physical world creates a smooth, bright, shiny, wide open road between you and the universe. It is a clear invitation that you are ready and willing to receive the guidance and apply it in your life.

Begin to think only positive, descriptive words for your developing intuitive abilities and take the negative words out of your experience. Instead of thinking negatively about yourself, begin thinking positively with thoughts such as:

"I am intuitive."

"I notice my intuition."

"I deeply trust my intuition."

"The spiritual world does exist and I am more and more aware of it."

"Of course that happened."

"I immediately notice synchronicity."

"I feel a deep knowing."

"I knew Spirit was with me when that happened."

"I am so proud of myself and my level of awareness."

Do not be ashamed that you sense and perceive more than those around you. They are only upset or afraid of the non-physical realms. Most will not have the same understanding of life that you obviously have. Allow yourself to stand up straight with your eyes bright with pride. You really can be respectful, compassionate, and kind knowing that you are a sacred being, but so are others no matter where they are at in their personal development. The clear steps are here for you to deliberately take charge of your body, emotions, thoughts, and life as you continue your sacred journey into your own soul.

You are a spirit in a spirit-filled environment. You are not separate from the non-physical realms. You are non-physical and physical at the exact same time. If you do not trust yourself first and foremost, you are transmitting a powerful signal that you do not trust the divine and sacred guidance either. This really is no more than a decision and a choice for you to decide to trust.

Stop Now and Notice Yourself with Fascination

Take a moment to honestly evaluate your level of trust. Is it there? Is it missing? Is it gone? When and where did it go? You are the only one with the power to decide to trust yourself.

Essential Points

• Your thoughts manifest your life.

• You are your thoughts.

• Your thoughts are directing everything.

• You are manifesting with your thoughts.

• You are an important link in the universe.

• You can be a weak link or a powerful creative link.

- Your mind is the Internet connecting into the universe.

- You are an electrical being in an electrical universe.

- One of your greatest purposes in life is to decide how you will use your power.

- Use your power for the greatest good or misuse it for power over others.

- Trust yourself and trust the divine and sacred. Be proud of your abilities.

Chapter 5

Your Emotions are Empowering Everything

"Nothing brings out the worst in another faster
than your focusing upon it. Nothing brings out the
best in another faster than your focusing upon it."

—Esther Hicks, *The Astonishing Power of Emotions*

I have been talking about your thoughts as dynamic electrical currents. Now let's discuss emotions. If thoughts are electrical frequencies of information, then emotions are the power behind them. The power behind your thoughts can be weak, strong, negative, or positive. The power of emotions can be present, or it can be nonexistent.

I asked my client to look down inside of his abdomen just above his belly button and look inside of the pain.

He quickly said, "How do I get rid of it?"

I asked that we try not to get rid of it just yet. I suggested, "Let's check in with the pain first in order to receive information about it."

He agreed, saying that made a lot of sense to him.

This client asked the pain multiple questions one at a time. He asked the questions I suggested and then asked some of his own questions. He did not move on to the next question until he noticed whatever picture or words popped into his thoughts or his mind's eye. There were heavy emotions hidden deep down inside of his solar plexus. The pain answered his questions. (More details about this later on in the book.)

Are You Reacting or Taking Action?

Every one of us has stuff. The human experience of life on earth seems to be full of stuff. Even people who are considered experts about some aspect of life all have their own stuff. It seems that no one gets through this human life without gathering some baggage along the way. The primary thing that makes all the difference in the world is this . . . It all depends on what you do with your stuff.

When you find yourself saying things like, "Why did I do that?" "What was I thinking?" "I wonder why I said what I said just now?" "Oh no, I did it again!" That sudden awareness is a signal for you to notice something about yourself. Catch yourself when your inner voice says those things inside of your head. Allow it to be a teaching moment just for you and about you. It is a positive awareness. It only has the possibility to become negative if you allow your negative behavior or negative thoughts to continue again and again. Get in charge of you and stop the negative dialogue. Take action and shift your awareness into: "I wonder what I need to learn right now?" Then take whatever pops into your mind. The pop will be the truth for you to learn.

Do not react to the world around you. Other people react based on the weight of the emotional load they are carrying within their body, energy field, and soul. When you find yourself reacting to people or events, you are not in your personal place of empowerment. When our emotions dominate our thoughts and our wisdom, we react to people, places, and moments.

Taking action is completely different. You are in charge of you. You are not flailing or floundering. The wise one within you assesses the situation, considers options, goals, and solutions. The wise one within you requests more information from the universe and unfolds intuitive guidance. All this can happen within a split second of earthly time. You are in grasp of the greater picture. You are not operating from raw emotions. You are the authority of you.

Eckhart Tolle talks about emotions in a lovely way. "Make it a habit to ask yourself: What's going on inside me at this moment? That question will point you in the right direction. But don't analyze, just watch. Focus your attention within. Feel the energy of the emotion. If there is no emotion present, take your attention more deeply into the inner energy field of your body. It is the doorway into Being."

Guilt, Confusion, Shame, Fear, Blame, Remorse, Judgment, Jealousy

Shame, guilt, fear, depression, grief, and other similar emotions have an intense sluggish, thick, sticky vibration. We even tend to call them "sickening emotions." The energy of these emotions in general are heavy, thick, and slow moving so they quickly become more physical. Each of these emotions, however, have their own type of sluggish vibration. Each of these individual emotions tend to congregate in certain areas of the human body, and eventually cause physical illness or a disease.For example, depression may tend to appear like a dark stocking cap on a person's head. When a person grieves the loss of someone or something very essential to them, it takes their breath away. Often, within three to four months, the grieving person will be diagnosed with lung cancer. Some people dealing with shame or remorse are so completely empty that you might find yourself looking past their rib cage into an empty cavern within their chest. It's as if their heart and lungs have disappeared. Another example is the feeling of shame or being shamed by someone. Shame creates not only a heavy burden, but it also drains the life out of an individual. That electrical vibration of shame clusters in the solar plexus just above your belly button because that is our energy center for our personal empowerment, our ability to be who we are meant to be as an individual.

Emotions are based on our thoughts and beliefs. They either empower our health and well-being or cause illness or life struggles. If your thoughts and the subsequent emotions are heavy burdens to you, then the energy is heavy and will burden your health and actions. I will show a chart later on showing where certain emotions tend to congregate in certain places or organs in our bodies.

But now I ask you, "Where are your happy emotions located in your body?" If you have positive or happy thoughts, the emotional fuel beneath those thoughts is fine, fast, buoyant, and sunny bright. The speed allows for a flowing current surging throughout your physical body. Your emotions are strong and, as a result, your body systems feel strong. You feel a sense of "all is well."

Mistakes and Secrets

Every single person on this earth has made mistakes. You are not alone even though you think you are. Notice what you do when you think of your mistakes. First, we go over it again and again. Sometimes we never stop going over it. Then we relive it, and by doing that we actually give it a life of its own. This repetition gives it life and also a portion of your "aliveness" remains in those moments of mistakes. When you repeat the scenario in your head, you inject that moment with more aliveness and so on.

What you can do now is decide to examine those mistakes in an entirely different manner. What I ask you to notice is this: Are you willing to consider noticing those mistakes from a different angle, or will you decide right now to hold on to them as you always have? Do not read on if you plan to beat yourself up for the remainder of your life.

Since you continued to read on, I will continue to discuss this with you.

1. If you have been viewing that moment again and again with the feelings of judgment, guilt, shame, anger, regret, or any other heavy, dark emotion, I ask that you stop reliving that moment again and again in the same old way.

2. Stop focusing on any other people, animals, or situations that were involved.

3. I ask you watch it from an entirely different angle. I ask you to shift from rehashing it in the same old way to studying only yourself in great detail.

4. Notice yourself as a soul. Notice your soul and not just a human being.

5. Notice that your soul is supposed to learn something from that situation.

6. Notice yourself without any judgment. Truly become more and more fascinated about you in the moment.

To be fascinated is to perceive something without judgment or criticism. Fascination is wanting to explore more details and more information about something. I ask that you learn all about you and how you turn this old moment into a positive piece of information. Be fascinated about who you are and what you are about and what makes you tick as the individual that you are now.

Secrets are not always about mistakes, and many mistakes are not a secret at all. Secrets do have their own electrical vibration but are very contained in what could be described as compressed, stuffed, boxed, sealed, protected, inaccessible, clenched, or locked away.

Again, thoughts and resulting emotions are electrical energy surges that gush and radiate throughout our body and then emanate outward into the world. This all takes place in less than a second and continues to happen nonstop throughout our days and nights. The opposite of that happens when we decide to keep a secret. Yes, it is a decision to keep something a secret. The flow is locked down and stashed away.

The secrets do not just remain in our head. While it crashes around in our head for a period of time, it also descends down into our throat area. It settles in the throat and often the thyroid because that is the portion of our body that represents expression. What are secrets about but the opposite of expressing something?

Stop Now and Notice Yourself with Fascination

What are the mistakes you have made in your life? Notice your secrets too. Only if you are willing, write each one down now. Do not focus on anyone else that is involved. Refuse to look at it in the ways you have always looked at it.

Look at each mistake through the eyes of your developing soul. Be interested in learning something about yourself without judgment.

Accidents are Not Accidental

My friend miscalculated the doorway as she quickly walked through it. She ran her right foot into the wood edging as she hurried to answer the phone. She could hear the little toe snap as it broke. Even accidents are not accidents. Car crashes, falling off a porch and shattering an arm, or falling off a ladder washing windows are just three simple examples of things we call accidents, and yet in the body, mind, and emotional connection, any of those incidents are bursting with symbolism and intuitive information because:

1. Our head is connected to our body to form one unit.

2. Our thoughts and emotions send perpetual information back and forth. What happens in our body or head powerfully symbolizes information on a very physical level.

3. There is meaning in everything around us . . . even with accidents.

Let's look at the symbolic information from my friend's broken toe. To discover the deeper meaning of a situation, you look at all the details involved in the moment. Each component of an accident is symbolic of what is happening. The recognizable details to notice in this simple example are:

Doorway, walking quickly, right foot, little toe, phone call.

I suggested that she might be struggling with a transition (doorway) from one thing to another. The transition is not going smoothly (hit the framework of the door). She might be struggling to take the right action or next step in life (right foot). She might feel conflicted or even slightly broken (broken little toe) about the changes in her life going too quickly (walking quickly) and not sure she wants to hear anymore (phone call).

When I mentioned the significance of the event, her mouth dropped open. "How did you know? That is exactly what is happening in my life."

I replied that I really had no idea since we had not talked for quite a while. I continued on, saying that there is meaning in everything around us and everything that happens to us. Listen carefully and notice the details when a person tells you something that has happened to them. Everything has symbolic meaning. Your physical life and your physical body are interconnected. Life always represents what is going on within your thoughts and your heart.

You No Longer Need to Remain a Victim

Hearing or thinking about the word "victim" sends potent waves of emotion through many of us. We give our power away in such tiny subtle ways, sometimes on a daily basis. Our power is also taken from us in more blatant, aggressive ways. Many people have experienced both in this lifetime.

I grew up in a very psychic family who expected kids to be clairvoyant and expected kids to see deceased family members. Nobody was taught any classes because the adults didn't speak of it at all. They just accepted that you perceived the non-physical world. They accepted it because they knew it existed right along with us in the living. Being intuitively aware does not mean being kind, however. My intuitive parents were abusive and cruel. We children were basically servants attending to all the needs of our mother, the house, and the farm.

We were drained of our power at such a young age before we had a chance to have any strength, let alone power. We were physically, mentally, and emotionally injured. We were bashed, shamed, belittled, and disgraced daily in so many ways. Some victims have had their power ripped from them through abuse, violence, or neglect. Many times this happens at a young age when we are more vulnerable. Children have not had a chance to experience a moment of empowerment yet.

Victims tend to live their lives based on the wants or needs of others and without thought of themselves. A victim struggles to say no to anyone or simply is unable to say no at all. A victim has lost their personal sense of who they really are, what they really like or love, what they want or need to do for themselves. Life is about everyone else, and they usually have little thought about having their own desires, requests, or wishes.

A long time ago, one of my counseling clients gave up a distinguished position as a soccer coach to take care of her elderly mother. She stopped communicating with her friends and colleagues and stopped contact with the outside world. She shared with me that when she resigned her position and moved in with her mother that her mother's dementia was already so advanced that she didn't even realize that my client was her daughter. My client quickly began describing herself more and more as a victim of these circumstances, as if she had no choice. In this example, the client did have multiple choices. She just could not see them or find them in her awareness.

I must discuss bullies now as well. A bully is a scary individual who often uses cruelty to intimidate and demean people nearby. I will admit that a bully can be ruthless and frightening but they can only do what they do when there is a victim nearby. The bully has radar-like sensors for a person who has been victimized. The radar picks up the behavior and body movements of the victim, but they also pick up the weakened electrical energy of the victim as well.

Here are the traits of a bully:

- A bully is rarely alone. He or she always has someone to back them up.
- A bully waits for an audience to witness their strength.

- A bully tests the potential victim in some way to make sure they will surrender to the abuse.

- A bully only continues if the victim shifts even more into victimization.

- A bully backs down if the victim stands their ground.

The bully is the weakest, most terrified individual in the room. They feel so low about themselves that they must smash everyone down around them to have any sense of their own strength. The bully lost most, if not all, of their power way before the heartless viciousness began. The bully was a raging victim way before the brutality began.

In the moment, we do not recognize that we are losing our power and sense of being a strong individual. You really and truly can still take your power back. It is never too late. One of our primary life purposes is to understand just how powerful we are meant to be. When we get a hint or a clue that we have been victimized or allowed ourselves to become victims, there are doable healing action steps. We can genuinely heal, remove, and release the old trauma that stripped our strength away. It is never too late to fill ourselves with the truth and energy of our personal empowerment. The encouraging news is there are healing methods later in this book to generate healing from trauma and suffering.

I read a story somewhere about a physician who wrote a prescription for a patient. That prescription stated, "Stop being a victim." This physician did not place a date on the prescription. He asked the patient to choose a date that she decided upon and then write the date on it herself. It was so much more dramatically powerful for the patient to write the date than for the physician to do it. Basically, it was her decision to take her power back. You do not need to have a prescription from a doctor to take the needed steps. Write your own prescription and give it a date for yourself!

Raymon Grace, a well-known dowser that I just love, said this in a course I took with him.

"Maybe the best way to eliminate bullies is to eliminate victims. A victim cannot be a victim unless they have an abuser or bully. The bully cannot be a bully unless they have a victim, so they attract each other. Life is a matter of choices. Either person can choose to be, or not be, a victim or bully. The bully is not likely to make that choice, so the victim can make it for them. The first step is to choose *not* to be a victim."

Stop Now and Notice Yourself with Fascination

Allow me to ask you this question: When did you lose your power? Take the most instant thought that bounded into your mind. Now write your own prescription and decide the date that it begins.

Do I Need to Forgive?

My answer is no! I never ask or even suggest that anyone needs to forgive themselves or forgive someone else. Are you shocked? I am absolutely adamant about never telling someone they need to forgive. This is such an emotional topic that I have had people jump up from their seats in my workshop screaming at me and bursting into tears. That is one example of how big this topic is to people.

If you are told to forgive before you have healed, you too will be furious. We humans cannot forgive until we have healed. Forgiveness comes naturally after the healing takes place. When an authentic and genuine healing happens, there is a permanent release and liberation from the pain and the painful moment. That does not mean the moment is wiped from our memory. It does not mean we forget it. It means that the raw emotion that pounds within us now becomes a neutral piece of information in our history and nothing more.

Do you see and feel that difference? We do not forget what happened, but we are no longer burdened with any emotion about it or the people involved. Forgiveness is the spontaneous result of your healing. Do not allow anyone to insist that you must forgive. You will achieve forgiveness when you have decided to heal and release the people and the events that happened. You are more and more in charge of you.

Are You an Empath? What that Really Means

Do you consider yourself an empath? If you say yes to that question, then you will probably go on to say that you pick up everyone's emotions. You immediately feel what the other person is feeling. You struggle to be in stores or public areas because you are so affected by the struggles that other people are going through. You struggle to watch the news on television. This empathic client has struggled for years.

Client: One of my questions is that my guides give me a veil regarding my family members. I have a younger brother going through a detrimental, difficult time. I have been trying to work with him energetically, but I keep taking on his energy. So I send it back to him. Then soon I feel like I am going to die, so I send it back again. I feel like I have a magnet inside of me.

TZ: Does this happen just with him or with lots of people?

Client: I do this with lots of people but especially him. I am aware that I do this. I check into my body and ask, "Is this mine?" and usually it is not mine. I am aware that I do this, so I practice checking in with my body and 99 percent of the time, it is not mine. Then I go about my day. I do not understand why this keeps happening?

TZ: There are multiple reasons. But first of all when you notice it, I want you to command and really mean it when you say it. "This is not mine. Out of me *now!*" Then feel like you are pushing it out. Always say the word now in your commands because spirit is wishy washy about time.

Number two. Your energy field is too porous. I want you to

run the toroidal field with your mind and your breath to work like a pumping mechanism. Do you believe that you can get in charge and stop taking on everyone's stuff?

Client: Yes, I believe it, but it keeps happening, so I doubt it now.

TZ: The energy field around your heart and back are very vulnerable. I want you to work with the toroidal field and do the steps to deliberately build up your field. (See the Toroidal field Steps). Also, command: "I am a powerful link in the system of the Universe. I am the brightest light to assist others and myself *now*."

Client: I always forget to use the word "now" and to command. I struggle with asking versus commanding.

TZ: Well, when I say "command," it is not about being the boss. It is about meaning it and feeling what I say. When many people pray there is no *umph* or deep feelings behind their words. It is very mechanical. When you feel powerful about your words to the universe, it sends out a stronger frequency, and the universe then picks up the information more readily. It is very mechanical. If we put out something vague, they have to respond in a like frequency that is vague.

Empaths are amazingly empathetic. The dictionary definition describes it as the ability to understand and to share the feelings of others. Yes, we intuitives need to understand the complex lives with struggles and heartaches that our fellow humans are suffering with. Empaths, and intuitives in general, are crippled due to attracting emotional people to them and then absorbing the emotions of others. If you identify as an empath, try to stay with me and hear me out before you slam the book shut. I want and hope to offer you a new viewpoint to consider and for you to take an entirely different action for others and for yourself. This person often experiences a draining effect when around other people.

Client: I was with my husband's cousin yesterday, and as soon as she left, everything came crashing down. I kept saying to myself yesterday, "I think she brought me down!" then I would say "No! Don't put that on her. It's not her." But it was like she sucked the life out of me and then it was like I was going down a tube!"

TZ: Now listen to your words. You are describing *exactly* what was happening with that woman. You are describing an intuitive wisdom coming to you, but you are not recognizing it as intuition. The word "vampire" came from somewhere, and in my opinion, it is from people realizing that they have been sucked dry by someone. Those people do not know that they can generate their own power. They become needy or a victim, and so they begin pulling from others. They are not doing this intentionally. They usually have no idea they have this effect on anyone. You can stop it from happening again, however.

Basically, you allowed it, but not on purpose. You were not aware you have the ability to stop it. And she probably was not aware either. Some people do this on purpose and deliberately. Also, many dead people continue to drain alive people too. If they did it when alive, they often continue to do this draining as a deceased person.

Client: Boy, I have a lot to learn.

TZ: Well, mostly I teach from the hard knocks that I have had. That is why I hope to get my information out to the world, so others do not suffer. Let's put this into action for yourself about this woman who drained you.

Call out to the Universe for your divine, sacred guide who specializes in cleansing filters to come forward and provide the cleansing filter for you. Command, "I bring me and only me back to me clean and clear through the filter provided for me from full name of the person. (More about this command later on.)

Client: It feels lighter. It is amazing how physically good this feels. I feel like I could do this all day, it feels so good.

TZ: I would also beg you to crank up your own energy with the toroidal field. You need to build up your own energy deliberately to be more and more in charge of you. That is deliberately running the rainbows and gold. (More on the toroidal field later.)

Empaths really are struggling because they are absorbing the emotional vibrations emanating from people around them. They are functioning as if they are dry sponges, mopping up all the sadness, heartache, and turmoil that ventures near them. They are merging with those negative emotions belonging to others and do not seem to be aware that they have a choice to continue to be empaths, or they can choose to get in charge of their own energy fields and save themselves.

Do not emotionally merge into or identify with people around you, and be careful to not take on their illnesses or suffering. Aligning with the emotions of others will force you into their emotional spectrum. Energetically merging with the struggles and heavy emotions of others will only add your personal emotions to the emotional energy for both of you. Your own body and your own life is simply merging and adding to the total energy of the suffering of humanity without healing you or others.

Take care of yourself first and foremost. Stop feeling everyone's suffering. There, I said it out loud. Feeling and merging into the suffering of others only adds more suffering to your life. You cannot lead yourself into health if you keep merging into other people's suffering, their life story, their shame or guilt. You will not heal or be an accurate intuitive if you take on and carry their emotions.

Dr. Norm Shealy and I were interviewed during a summit gathering. During his interview he states, "Every thought is a prayer." I got chills as he said those words.

Dr. Shealy went on to discuss his own self-care. "I am inevitably interested in protecting my true life's energy from chaos . . . It's not worth wasting my life energy on." He continued, "The transcendent will of the soul is extremely important. The transcendent will is paying attention to our personal soul's connection."

It is your choice now . . . Merge with the suffering around you or become a more dazzling, illuminating escort, pointing and guiding others out of their darkness into their own very personal power.

Stop Now and Notice Yourself with Fascination

Notice what is happening within you as we discuss topics such as forgiveness and also suffering. Notice without any judgment.

Essential Points

- Your emotions either fuel your thoughts or take the fuel away.
- Mistakes are moments to learn something vital about yourself and your soul.
- Secrets are emotions clenched and sealed within your body.
- Negative emotions are thick and slow, causing physical illness in certain locations in the body.
- Positive emotions are light, fine, and fast, creating a healthier body.
- Everything has meaning, even accidents.
- Visualizing sends a strong signal to the universe.
- You no longer need to remain a victim.
- Bullies are the most damaged victims.
- Empaths understand the misery of others but must not merge with it.
- Heal first, then forgiveness will arrive naturally.

Chapter 6

Intuitively Know Your Own Energy Field

"Intuition goes before you, showing you the way.
Emotion follows behind, to let you know when
you go astray. Listen to your inner voice."

—Anthon St. Maarten, *Divine Living*

The universe and all living things within it are electrically alive. You and I are electrical and so is everyone else. Your body and organs function electrically. Our nervous system is basically tiny wires for electrical bits of information to surge back and forth from brain to body parts and organs then back to the brain. An electric spark sets off every single beat of your heart. First responders use paddles to shoot electric jolts at our heart to stimulate its beating again. Many medical tests such as MRIs, CAT Scans, EEG, and EKG are electrically-based tests because humans are electrical.

Your Aura is Your Soul

Your soul is the electrically vibrating aliveness within the body you are dwelling within at this time. Your soul is much larger than your body. The cords to our appliances are surrounded with insulation to contain the electrical power and funnel it from the electrical source to the appliance. Our skin, however, does not hold the electrical power in like rubber cords do, so that enlivened power extends outward beyond the skin. That electrical vibration inhabits every cell of your body, and at the same time, it exudes out beyond the skin.

People are not the only ones with an aura. When alive, animals, birds, fish, trees, plants, grass, and the earth all have auras. For example, my solid black cat used to play by jumping into the white bathtub. Even though she was a "black cat" she would fill the tub with her shimmery, bright-green aura. So I would always tell people that I have a green cat. If you look at a group of trees, especially in the spring, you will see clear energy shooting outward at all kinds of angles as they wake up for summer. I have witnessed rainbows rising up out of the ground in New Zealand because the earth itself is alive and has an aura.

The aura is the electrically alive eternal soul. It enters into a body and the individual lives their physical life. At the time of death, the aura then begins to separate from each cell until it finally leaves the physical body completely. I have witnessed this departure happening in many different ways. One man's soul lifted up while remaining in a horizontal way parallel to his body. When his soul rose about two feet above his body, I perceived thousands of threads between the soul body and the physical body. Then the threads became thinner and thinner and finally released from the body. I have also seen the soul actually sit up and look around before rising upward. My friend's cat was in his dying process. As it happened, I saw sparkles exit from the base of his neck as his aliveness rose up and out of his ill body.

Your Aura Colors are Information

It seems that everyone wants and hopes to see auras. Most people are unconsciously seeing them though they do not realize it. The primary reason that people think they are failing to see auras is that they are looking for something thick and dense that holds quite still. This, in fact, is the direct opposite of how the aura behaves. For example, when you are exhausted, your aura will shrink back close to the skin. When you are happy and alert your aura is large, bright, and translucent. For example, when you drive around a curve and suddenly a stunning mountain range stands before you and you are swept with delight. Your energy field instantly expands and heightens. Those positive emotions sent electrical currents throughout your body and then outward into your field.

Earlier, I discussed how powerful your thoughts are and how your emotions either fuel or weaken the power of each thought. Well, the aura displays exactly the truth of what is going on within your thoughts, emotions, and your physical body. The aura itself is the electrical extension of what is happening within each person. The aura fluctuates constantly with each thought and each emotion you have. The aura and the colors of the aura are simply and truthfully information. What shines out beyond the skin is happening within us.

To see your own aura, you must first make your eyes feel relaxed and even lazy. If you wear glasses or contacts, you might remove them to practice. Have a blank and neutral colored wall behind you. Do not try hard to see it. Look into a large mirror and look at the area above your head and shoulders. Look more at the wall than your head. Allow your eyes to relax and partially close in a sleepy way. Notice the air about two to three inches above your head and shoulders. Do not try to perceive any color yet. Just notice that the air seems lightly thicker or slightly wavy.

Notice how far the thicker air seems to extend above your head. Now imagine, yes, imagine and pretend that you are sending a certain color upward from your head. Notice and be playful with yourself. Notice the energy above your head when you are exhausted and when you are feeling great and alive. Because the aura moves with us, it will draw close to the skin when we are depleted and will extend outward, large and brighter when we feel refreshed and invigorated.

As you grow more comfortable and trust yourself you will also notice that different organs or sections of your body emit different colors. You will also begin to notice that the shade and thickness of each color gives you even more information about that area of your body.

On the next page you will find a list of colors and the meaning that vibrates within the spectrum of that color. You might notice that each color has positive and not-so-positive meanings. Notice more detail about colors than just the general color. Noticing the following will lead you to recognize more information that the color really means.

Take note of these details as you notice colors:

- Location of each color within or outside of your body. If the color is within the body, notice the organ, chakra, or section of the body where the color is located.

- Shade of each color.
  - Bright and shiny means the positive quality of that color.
  - Darker, dim, brownish or grayish means the more negative qualities of each color.

- Movement or lack of movement.
  - Flowing out from you means you are sending it out to others or to the world.
  - Flowing inward to you means you are receiving it from someone or somewhere.
  - Lack of movement might signify that an area in your body is struggling or blocked.

- Density or thickness of each color:
  - Thin, transparent, shimmery means health.
  - Thick, heavy, opaque, solid means the area is not vital, low functioning.

Aura Colors and Meaning	
Red	Cellular health, energy, high temper, movement, extroversion
Light Red	Nervous, impulsive, passion, eroticism, sexuality, love
Dark Red	Willpower, masculinity, rage, courage, suffering, leadership
Pink	Femininity, longings, sensitivity, emotional, softness
Brown	Egotism, addiction, disease, earthiness, unloving
Orange	Active intelligence, confident, expressive, warmth, joy of life, sex
Orange-Red	Taking action, pride, vanity, idealism, desire
Orange-Yellow	Sharp intellect, quick wit, industrious
Yellow	Clear and active thinking, intellectual abilities
Dark Yellow	Timidity, thriftiness, restrictions, control needs
Gold	Devotion, higher inspiration, meditative state, authority, creativity
Forest Green	Abundance, harvest, deep level of healing
Green	Growth, change, nature, devotion, neutral state, healing, harmony
Light Green	Sympathy, direct, possible deceit or lying
Blue	Introversion, solitude, truth, devotion to spirit, wisdom, prayer, writing
Light Blue	Soft, reserved, religious, struggle to mature
Indigo	Healing ability, immersed in work, morality, spirituality, mediumship
Turquoise	Giving love to others in a healing capacity, expansion
Lavender	Mysticism, magic, overbearing, obsessions
Violet	Intuition, art, creativity, supernatural, imagination
Clear White	Eternal, forever, Godlike
Milky White	Spirituality, higher consciousness, physical pain
Silver	Love about the Great Mother
Black	Protection, shielding, detached from senses, negative interference
Gray	Low energy, depression, sadness, physical illness

Stop Now and Notice Yourself with Fascination

What colors do you feel the best while wearing? What colors do you love to have around you? This is interesting information about yourself.

Thoughts and Emotions Affecting the Body

Your body is not separate from your emotions or your thoughts. Your head and body are actually one unit. Your thoughts and feelings end up in your physical body. Positive thoughts and their subsequent emotions disperse fast and clear throughout the body creating vitality and cellular health. Negative thoughts and emotions are slow, sticky, and sluggish. That vibrational slowness tends to allow it to gather rather than flow. Due to its sluggish, listless movement, negative thoughts and emotions tend to clump or congregate in the body. As emotional energy continues to gather in a location, a physical struggle, illness or disease will begin to develop.

It is interesting that certain emotions congregate in certain organs or sections of our body. For example, when responsibility for something or someone weighs heavier and heavier, then that emotion will usually congeal in the shoulders and lower vertebra of the neck around the cervical six and cervical seven. Another example, under all physical pain is always unresolved emotional pain. The location of the physical pain in the body will then tell you even more detailed information about it.

Do you realize, however, if we are powerful enough to make ourselves ill, we are powerful enough to make ourselves well.

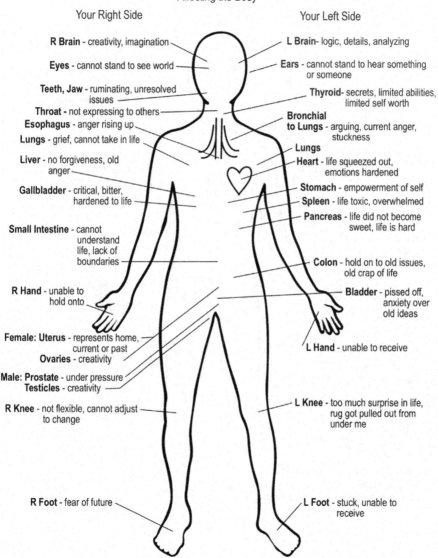

Diagram - Thoughts and Emotions
Affecting the Body

Your Right Side

Your Left Side

R Brain - creativity, imagination

L Brain - logic, details, analyzing

Eyes - cannot stand to see world

Ears - cannot stand to hear something or someone

Teeth, Jaw - ruminating, unresolved issues

Thyroid - secrets, limited abilities, limited self worth

Throat - not expressing to others

Bronchial to Lungs - arguing, current anger, stuckness

Esophagus - anger rising up

Lungs

Lungs - grief, cannot take in life

Heart - life squeezed out, emotions hardened

Liver - no forgiveness, old anger

Stomach - empowerment of self

Gallbladder - critical, bitter, hardened to life

Spleen - life toxic, overwhelmed

Pancreas - life did not become sweet, life is hard

Small Intestine - cannot understand life, lack of boundaries

Colon - hold on to old issues, old crap of life

R Hand - unable to hold onto

Bladder - pissed off, anxiety over old ideas

Female: Uterus - represents home, current or past

Ovaries - creativity

L Hand - unable to receive

Male: Prostate - under pressure

Testicles - creativity

R Knee - not flexible, cannot adjust to change

L Knee - too much surprise in life, rug got pulled out from under me

R Foot - fear of future

L Foot - stuck, unable to receive

Be Your Own Medical Intuitive
©2021 Tina M. Zion

Diagram - Thoughts and Emotions
Affecting the Body

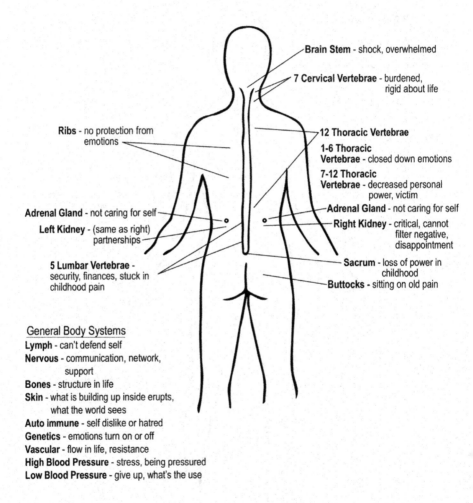

Brain Stem - shock, overwhelmed

7 Cervical Vertebrae - burdened, rigid about life

Ribs - no protection from emotions

12 Thoracic Vertebrae

1-6 Thoracic Vertebrae - closed down emotions

7-12 Thoracic Vertebrae - decreased personal power, victim

Adrenal Gland - not caring for self

Left Kidney - (same as right) partnerships

Adrenal Gland - not caring for self

Right Kidney - critical, cannot filter negative, disappointment

5 Lumbar Vertebrae - security, finances, stuck in childhood pain

Sacrum - loss of power in childhood

Buttocks - sitting on old pain

General Body Systems

Lymph - can't defend self
Nervous - communication, network, support
Bones - structure in life
Skin - what is building up inside erupts, what the world sees
Auto immune - self dislike or hatred
Genetics - emotions turn on or off
Vascular - flow in life, resistance
High Blood Pressure - stress, being pressured
Low Blood Pressure - give up, what's the use

Stop Now and Notice Yourself with Fascination

Notice your body and notice the signals it is sending to you right now. For example, where is there tightness, pain, stiffness, or swelling? Notice your own emotions within your body. Are they making you ill or well at this moment?

Essential Points

• Your aura is the visible part of your soul that cannot be contained beneath your skin.

• Your aura is alive and fluctuates with every thought and emotion.

• Colors are not just colors. They are waves of information.

• Your body and your head are one unit. What happens in your thoughts happen in your body.

• Certain emotions tend to congeal in certain areas of the body and eventually cause illness.

• If our thoughts and emotions make us physically ill, then we are capable to make ourselves well.

Chapter 7

Intuitively Get in Charge of Your Energy Field — Power Up!

"Your energy body is your personal frequency.
It is as unique to you as your fingerprint."

—Catherine Carrigan, *The Little Book of Breathwork*

I was talking to a friend, describing and guiding her to scan her own energy field. As she followed my instructions, she said with alarm in her voice, "My energy field is totally wimpy!"

I titled this section *Power Up!* because one of my dear clients, S.B., said it is vitally important to discuss with the readers how powerful we are. She feels that "Power Up" describes it well. Few people are aware that we humans have the ability to manage, supervise, and direct our own energy field as well as affect the energy fields of others.

Scientific research continues to find that energy follows human thought. Can you truly allow that to soak in? Research has found that we humans can move pinballs from thousands of miles away with our focused thoughts. Human thoughts can alter material objects in the physical world. Energy practitioners and medical intuitives use these discoveries as the foundation of their work. Since energy follows human thought, then each thought we think is a powerful, living thing with substance and force!

Setting our intent simply means humans have the ability to intensely focus our thoughts. Focused thought literally sends a well-defined electrical frequency from the person's brain and body outward into the Universe. Be much more careful with your thoughts. Get in charge of your thoughts and do not let them be in charge of you. You have the ability to create an intent more powerful than you could ever dream. Use that power of focused thought to create well-being for yourself first and foremost.

As I have mentioned in my other books, I ask people to stop protecting themselves with energetic bubbles, crystal-egg shapes, or even beautiful walls. When someone creates any type of protection around them, even if it is crystalline, it first generates most often during a time of fear suspicion, jealousy, or similar emotions. Because the emotion of fear is so intense, all we really end up creating is an even stronger bubble of fear around us. Fear has a much stronger frequency than protection does. As a result, rather than protection, we cause more fear to envelop us.

Does that make sense to you? We meant to create protection, but fear is so dense, concentrated, and opaque that we create a sticky grayish energy around us instead. Not only are we not protecting ourselves, but we essentially created more of an interference around us. That thickening shield around you based in fear deeply interferes with the natural flow of your energy but also interferes with receiving the positive wonders in life.

Over time, our fear causes the wall of protection to become a thickened barrier. This barrier does not keep out the negative. In fact, it attracts negativity and diminishes our ability to receive the positive in life.

Instead of building walls out of fear, use the power of your focused thought, known as intent, to build your personal energy field from inside of your body and allow it to shine outward. Deliberately enrich your own energy, first inside of you, and then allow that richness to shine out to all the world and beyond. Build up and power up your energy on a daily basis when you are feeling good. Do not wait until you are in a fearful situation and end up putting a barrier around you. You want to constantly work with your personal energy field to become brighter and more powerful. The bright sparkles of who you are naturally meant to be actually repel the negativity.

You are more than your body. You are a physical body, but you are also the energy field of your soul. You need to attend to both at the same time. When you suffer from working so hard or painful situations or disappointments in life your body takes a hit, but with any emotional hit, your energy field takes a hit as well. This is because you are both physical and energetic at the exact same time.

Most of us take a shower every day because our body picks up dust; we feel sweaty or a bit sticky as the day goes on. Tensions and feelings come and go, and some stay as we lug around unresolved feelings. As we interact with people around us, we notice their tensions and feelings too. Some emotions from other people stick to us and some suddenly shoot at us like sharp arrows out of nowhere. While our thinking mind tries to sort out the tension or conflict, our energy field has taken some of those emotional strikes at the same time.

As life continues to happen, your energy field sends and receives energy such as love and appreciation, or anger and irritation, and the full spectrum of emotions people have. As the day goes on, your thoughts, emotions, and reactions to events affect your energy field. But at the same time, the people interacting with you affect your energy field as well. For example, if someone is intensely jealous or irritated or angry with you, their energy emits a sharp flash of energy that comes your way. Their negative energy can alter your energy when it thrusts toward you, and at the same time, your energy affects others too.

This can happen even when people do not mean any harm to you. A burst of emotion inside of a human extends outward to the focus of their emotions. Your energy does the same thing if you interact emotionally with others as well.

This exchange of energy surging back and forth is natural, and it happens constantly in positive ways and in negative ways. This movement and extension of human thought energy is also called "telepathy," or the sharing of information energetically between people. Our energy fields also extend outward to others when we care about someone and when we love others. There is so much more going on in the non-physical realms than the physical realm. We are so much more than a body with a thinking head on top of it!

Just like a hot shower or a soothing bath, your energy field needs some daily care as well. First you need to look, feel, and notice your energy field. Here are the basic steps to scan your own energetic field.

First, remember three key intuitive concepts . . .

- Intuitive awareness will always seem like you are imagining, pretending, and making it all up.

- Always take the *pop* of awareness that leaps into your mind.

- Do not work hard or put any effort into intuition. Passively notice whatever you notice with fascination.

Human Form to Record Your Personal Scans

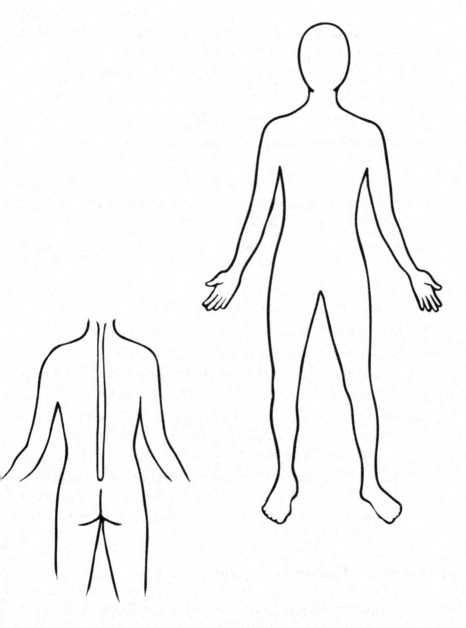

Be Your Own Medical Intuitive
©2021 Tina M. Zion

Steps to Scan Your Energy Field

1. Shift your thoughts to scanning yourself without judgment or criticism. Only move forward with increased fascination about knowing yourself on a deeper level.

2. Direct your thoughts to focus on the alive energy surrounding your physical body.

3. Be fascinated and allow yourself to trust the intuitive you.

4. Imagine hypersensitive antennae at the end of your focused thoughts.

5. Notice that your energy does indeed extend past your skin 360 degrees all around you in every direction. Do not forget your backside and under your feet.

6. Allow the sensors to notice how far your energy extends outward from your skin.

7. Notice the feel, the color, and the look of your energy around the outside of your body.

8. Notice where your field is rich with energy.

9. Look for areas that seem, feel, or look different than the rest of your field. Look for areas that are thin, weak, dim, open, torn, discolored, or any tunnels or depressions.

10. It will always feel like your imagination, but look for objects or impressions of objects in your field such as: dark cords, knives, arrows, or any objects in general.

11. Draw with colored markers or pencils on the human form provided here. This form is located in the back of the book for you to print copies to document the intuitive information you perceive.

Your Personal Toroidal Field—The Flow of Your Soul

Many spiritual teachers train people to only direct a portion of their energy field. Many instructors discuss bringing your energy down and into the crown of your head. Some say to bring it up from the ground. Either way, it is only a portion of what it takes to power up our energy field to its finest and most powerful.

The human toroidal energy field is a smooth, full cycle of energy deliberately running in and around you in both directions. Your personal energy field needs to flow both up and down, but in a smooth, interactive movement exactly like a fountain in a pond. A fountain is simply a pump. It draws water up from the pool until the pump fills so full it shoots upward into the air then falls back into itself without any effort.

Science has recognized that the human energy field moves just like a fountain in a pond. Science calls this the human toroidal field. When I first came across a scientist's diagram of the toroidal field, I almost jumped out of my chair with surprise! I saw a diagram showing a fountain of energy flowing through a human. This is exactly how I have been seeing human energy for decades, and here is science stating the same thing.

This fountain formation was exactly the way I perceive energy flowing within people who are feeling exceptionally well physically, mentally, and emotionally! I could not believe that some scientists "think" that human energy moves in the same way that I have intuitively witnessed for years! Do you also remember, earlier in this book I mentioned that science has also discovered that energy follows human thought?

You need to realize. Believing it will put you more in charge of you.

Here is a simplified diagram showing the correct direction for you to take charge and instruct your toroidal field to flow. Please note, this not illustrating a barrier around you. This is showing only the up and down flow of your field.

Diagram – Human Toroidal Field

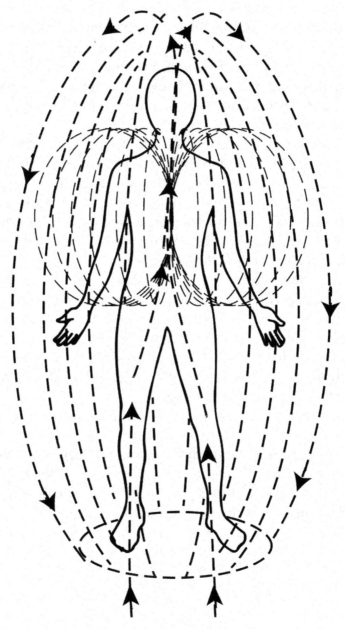

Be Your Own Medical Intuitive
©2021 Tina M. Zion

Steps to Repair and Heal Your Toroidal Field

Let's summarize before moving on. You have just examined the outer area of your energy field, recorded, and drew images on the human form that you noted regarding:

- Colors
- Brighter areas
- Weaker, dim, or thin areas
- Openings such as tears, holes, tunnels
- Foreign objects
- Anything else that popped into your awareness

You did not work hard at it, and you allowed perceptions to simply pop into your awareness. Remember, it will always feel as if you just imagined it. Go with whatever your awareness brings you. Trust whatever leaps into your awareness. You might find that your field is rich with energy, or full in some areas yet weak in others. Any type of weakened condition indicates the need for immediate action to bolster the natural protection that your energy field provides for you. If you sense any type of dark object in your field, feel your own empowerment and, with your thoughts, remove the object and send it up into the Light. You will then specifically fill that particular location with the toroidal field steps of rainbows, gold, diamonds, violet flame, and love.

It is about Powering *Up!* It is not about placing a barrier around you. It is about shining from the inside outward. It is your personal power, and it needs to be overflowing outward to the world. Now, you are realizing more and more that you have the ability to direct your energy field. Just by thinking about it in specific, focused ways, your energy will naturally follow your directives. I love it when science, intuitives, energy healers, and alternative health professionals find truth and come together with like minds.

Look at the drawing of the toroidal as you read the steps to deliberately direct your toroidal energy field in a precise manner. Imagine your energy field responding and flowing in this manner.

Deliberately take charge of your energy and practice right now.

1. Begin by simply breathing in your normal pattern, but this time notice all the sensations of inhaling. Focus on inhaling. Feel the breath entering into your nose, throat, and chest. Notice all the physical sensations of cool air coming in, touching the back of your throat, then quickly warming as it enters your chest.

2. Continue breathing normally, and at the same time, *imagine* that you are also inhaling up through the soles of your feet and inhaling through your nose or mouth.

3. Keep breathing into your feet. With each inhalation, imagine vibrant rainbows, sizzling gold, and diamond-like sparkles quickly rising into you. Continue to imagine rainbows, gold, and diamond-like sparkles completely filling your body so full that the energy rushes outward from every inch of your skin until you look like a bright lightbulb shining out and filling the room.

4. With your thoughts, deliberately fill any weakened areas, places where objects were located, openings, etc.

5. Now imagine that you are so full that the energy shoots out the top of your head and up into the cosmos as high as you can imagine.

6. Continue to breathe through the soles of your feet but now add a combination of rainbows, electrified gold, and sparkling diamonds.

7. Now your shine is even brighter and more robust.

8. Now send the vibrant rainbows, gold, and diamonds into each weakened area that you found in your field earlier. Fill every single place around you. You are repairing and healing your body and energy field now.

9. You are more and more in charge of you as you Power *Up!*

10. Then, like a fountain, your energy rises high up, making a powerful connection and link into the cosmos.

11. With no effort on your part, allow the cosmos to shower goodness down into you. It is your choice to receive it or not. You must deliberately allow your body and energy field to receive its abundance.

12. The cosmos gives back to you by flowing into your body and energy field and back into the earth and then, like a pumping fountain, up into your body and field again and again.

13. Practice until you can generate your internal and external fountain in just a few seconds. The rainbow vibration is cleansing and healing. Gold and diamonds are precious and repel the negative.

14. Finish by imagining standing inside of an intense, dazzling energy of violet fire.

15. Remember—your entire body becomes a pumping mechanism, exactly like a fountain in a park. Practice and playfully practice some more.

16. Remember also—You are not creating a barrier around you. You are gleaming from the inside of you then outward to the world.

The more you attend to your field on a daily basis, the more you will feel energized, secure, and alert. The more you do this daily, the faster and smoother it will happen. Run your toroidal field first thing in the morning and again at bedtime. Run your toroidal field swiftly all throughout your day. You will feel and know the difference in yourself.

Stop Now and Notice Yourself with Fascination

What is it like at this moment to notice yourself as a flowing electrical soul energy?

Explore the feelings of being more in charge of who you are meant to be. Is it uncomfortable or does it feel freeing?

Essential Points

- You are more than your body. You are also the energy field of your soul.

- The thoughts and emotions of both yourself and others affect your energy field.

- Your field should never be wimpy.

- You are in charge of your energy field to keep it empowered on a daily basis.

- Know yourself more completely. Scan your field instantly in 360 degrees around you.

- Repair and heal your energetic field daily. It is a great part of who you are.

- Do not create barriers with your field. Shine from the inside outward.

Chapter 8

Intuitively Communicate with Your Own Physical Body

"All mental illness is some form of *external* searching. Mental health is inner peace."
—Helen Schucman, *A Course in Miracles*

We have covered how to intuitively know your own energy field in a more detailed way. We then discussed how to get more in control and in charge of your energy field and the excellence of directing your toroidal field. Now we are discussing you at the physical level—your physical body and how to receive clearer, more accurate information regarding it. Your body speaks to you and is sending you important information.

People who attend my medical intuition live workshops or purchase my recorded course online come from a wide spectrum of backgrounds. Many of them have no idea where their internal organs are located or how they work, and still they yearn to do medical intuition for themselves or for others. At the other end of this spectrum lies physicians, nurse practitioners, physical therapists, and an array of other highly skilled medical professionals. Everybody sits together and readily shares their experiences. This happens because these people do share a common goal to become more intuitively aware of the human body. Others want to become more aware of different animals' physical bodies. But each individual yearns to receive intuitive wisdom about their health as well.

I have created the most basic, simple chart of the human anatomy. My goal for you is to learn the general location of your primary organs such as the gall bladder or the spleen. This is not for you to diagnose your issues but to take note of what organs you might be perceiving as you scan your own physical body.

Medical intuition for oneself is not really about diagnosing yourself. This is about receiving detailed, multifaceted intuitive information about your body, how it is doing well, or how and where it is ill or struggling. It is also about finding the causes of your struggles and how to heal and release them. We are, indeed, our own healer even as healers assist us in so many ways.

Simple Anatomy Chart – Front

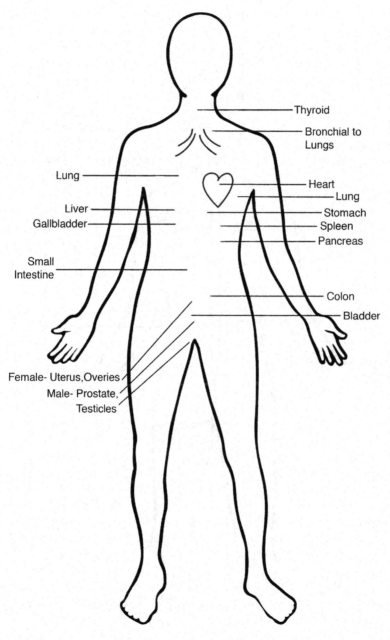

Thyroid

Bronchial to Lungs

Lung

Heart
Lung

Liver
Gallbladder

Stomach
Spleen
Pancreas

Small Intestine

Colon

Bladder

Female- Uterus,Overies
Male- Prostate,
Testicles

Be Your Own Medical Intuitive
©2021 Tina M. Zion

Simple Anatomy Chart – Back

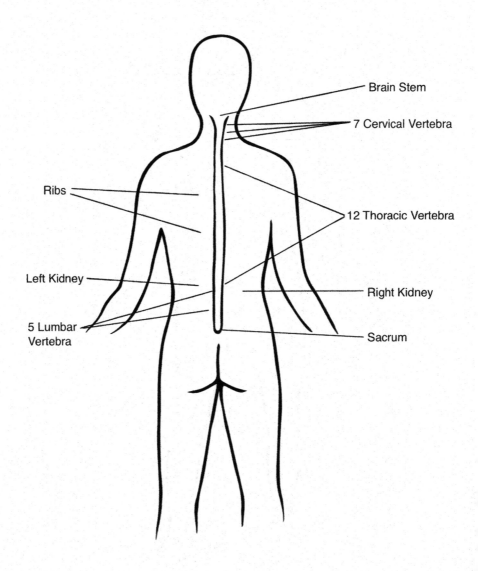

Brain Stem

7 Cervical Vertebra

Ribs

12 Thoracic Vertebra

Left Kidney

Right Kidney

5 Lumbar
Vertebra

Sacrum

Be Your Own Medical Intuitive
©2021 Tina M. Zion

Scan Your Body Like an X-Ray

When I discuss our human ability to literally look within a human body similar to an X-ray machine, people either do not believe it, they are excited to learn to do it, or they are so blown away they cannot find their words to describe their reactions. When I guide you in the following steps, you also might find this so simple that there must be more to it. Let's begin by discussing the simple anatomy and where our primary body parts are located.

Your thoughts are a powerful creative force. Energy naturally follows thought. Science has determined that is true. We humans have no idea how powerful thoughts really are. Look at your life right now. What you have and what you don't happens within your thinking mind first. The universe then follows the lead of your thought energy.

The following thoughts create a stronger energy signature: *I am intuitively skilled and more aware than ever before. I think, and the universe follows my energy. I really am able to scan my energy field and my physical body with interest and fascination. It will always and forever feel like my imagination. It will never stop feeling like my imagination, but it is deeply real.* Can you feel the difference as you read these words?

Your thoughts are powerful, and you are a powerful intuitive receiver. So far, this is what you have already accomplished with the guidance of this book:

- Created a focused intent to look outward and into your energy field.

- You have already directed and are training your energy to flow in the direction of the toroidal field.

- Your thoughts and skills are increasing in power.

- You are trusting only what *pops* into your awareness. Everything else is your thinking mind.

Your brain is only the computer. Your mind tells your computer brain where to go, what to do, and when to do it. Get in charge of your brain and your thoughts now. You can send yourself into a dreamy place when you choose. You can then feel a sense of settling downward, just a small amount, and begin to feel soft inside. The result is intentionally slowing down, feeling dreamy, and a slight downward softening sensation. You will know when you are more in sync with the intuitive channel of the Universe. You are deliberately tuning into your computer brain to become in sync with this intuition channel.

The accurate medical intuitive then hones their thought energy into a decisive laser beam and directs that beam inward. The medical intuitive then directs the laser beam even more precisely, going past the skin and into your own physical body. The area of your body that draws your attention will pull the laser beam towards itself.

Your hypersensitive laser beam is real. Your thoughts just created it and the laser beam energy will follow your precise and powerful thoughts. They clearly notice everything without any work.

One key point to remember: when you make that contact with your physical body, you may perceive a photo-like image or you may perceive a vague image. Simply stop, watch, and wait. The wait is usually only a few seconds. I wait because intuition is a gentle, passive movement. Receiving is the flow of information coming through your intuitive sensors and into your awareness. It is not about trying or pushing or working hard. It is about gentle acceptance and the gentle process of receiving.

You think you will remember everything, but you will not remember it for long because you will be in a light altered state of mind. Make copies of the human form. Use colored markers or pencils and a pen to write down messages that guides will give to you. Draw whatever you are noticing in your physical body and your energy field.

Basic Steps to Scan Your Body

1. Notice, instruct, and supervise your thoughts.

2. Gain more control by catching your old ways of thinking.

3. Instruct your thoughts to focus on the positive power they hold.

4. Concentrate your thoughts like a laser beam or like a flashlight on the highest beam.

5. Think and imagine your beam is hypersensitive, noticing and receiving everything without judgment.

6. Focus and create your laser beam.

7. Send your beam of awareness inside your body simply by thinking about doing that.

8. Begin with any location to which you were guided to go. Receive information for that area. Then move to the next.

9. Take note of everything that *pops* into your awareness.

10. Notice details and location of: your thoughts that pop, your mind's eye, colors, textures, images, symbols, pictures, guides, messages, smells, taste.

11. Go into areas of your body that feel good and healthier to you. Scan all around those areas. Take only the *pops*.

12. Also go into specific areas of your body that you are struggling with. Take the *pops* here as well. Use only your hypersensitive sensors to notice.

13. Document all details that come into your awareness on the human body form. You can make multiple copies for your future scans.

Each of us learns and thinks in different ways. Some learn more in images or sounds, and some learn more from lists and words. I include a list of body sections and body organs for you to print out and record your scans as well as the human body form to draw your personal scans. The choice is yours. You might feel best if you draw and write on the human form, or you might like to write descriptive words on the list below. You will also find all the different forms and steps in the back of the book to print out, if you want.

List of Body Sections and Organs to Guide Your Scans

- General View and First Impressions
- Aura/Energy Field
- Head
    Brain
    Face/Sinus
    Eyes
    Ears
    Jaw/Teeth
- Throat/Neck/Thyroid Gland
- Shoulders/Arms/Hands
- Chest
    Bronchial Tubes to Lungs
    Heart (slightly left of center)
    Breasts—male/female
- Upper Abdomen
    Stomach (center)
    Gallbladder (upper right side)
    Liver (upper right side)
    Spleen (upper left side)
    Pancreas (left side)
- Lower Abdomen
    Colon (across abdomen and down lower left side)
    Small Intestines (throughout lower abdomen)
    Female Ovaries (right and left sides)
    Female Uterus (Lower center abdomen)
    Bladder (lower center in pelvic area)
    Male Prostate (center behind bladder)
- Hips
- Legs
    Knees
    Ankles
    Feet
- Back
    Spine

Kidneys (right and left side above waistline)
Adrenal Glands (sits on top of each kidney)
Buttocks
- General Body Systems:
  Blood Vessels
  Bones
  Lymph
  Muscles/tendons
  Nerves
  Skin

Stop Now and Notice Yourself with Fascination

Allow your body to honestly speak to you or give you images. It has a great deal to say.

Essential Points

- Your thoughts are a powerful creative force.

- Energy naturally follows thought.

- Begin to realize how powerful your thoughts really are.

- Yes, you are able to look inside of your body like an X-ray machine.

- We are our own healer even as healers assist us in so many ways.

- You are not diagnosing as you scan yourself. You are receiving multifaceted intuitive information.

Chapter 9

Intuitively Communicate with the Universe

"Be bold and mighty forces will come to your aid."
—Johann Wolfgang von Goethe

You are not separate from the Universe. You are literally co-creating with the Universe every second of every day and every night. You can either be a weak link in the system or a powerful link. It is totally up to you.

I continue to hear that talking to God or guides does not result in answers or responses to people's prayers. Mentoring clients describe how they struggle to understand why they are not receiving spirit guidance in their healing work. They feel deeply that the guides, or the Universe, are not there for them. They only hear silence and often feel abandoned. People are trying so hard to heal themselves and others. When they get silence or fuzzy responses, they frequently want to give up. Many people do give up and stop altogether.

As we have discussed earlier, science shows that energy follows human thoughts. Think about this because it is key to your success as an intuitive . . .

Since it is true that your thoughts have substance and go out into the Universe, then it must also be true that one must launch the most exact, precise words when praying, or asking questions, talking to God or to your guides. I cannot emphasize this or accentuate this enough as an absolute crucial key to your success. You must use precise words that depict specifically what you are saying or asking God, Source, or your guides, or nothing can happen!

Like does attract like. That is a common spiritual message that makes sense to most of us. It is the same regarding communication with the non-physical realms. Guides are very literal about communication because it is energy, and they can only respond at the energetic level at which you form your requests to them.

Words You Use Makes All the Difference

I spend a great deal of time in mentoring sessions pointing out words and also phrases that are vague or actually mean the opposite of what you think you are asking guides to do. The mentoring clients and I then work together to figure out the best wording, to send the clearest signal, in order to get the best response from our guides.

Computers are based on using key words and also commands. To find anything, you need to type in the exact key words before the computer can take you to the correct place you want to go. It is exactly the same for our statements and requests to the Universe. If you are using nondescript words, then you get nonsensical, nondescript answers in return.

Your thoughts create your world by attracting or repelling objects, belongings, events, or relationships. Your thoughts attract or repel communication with the Universe. You are not repelling guides. You are generally preventing clear answers because of the energy of the words you are using. A good example is a question such as, "Can you help me?" You may actually get a "yes" but then silence. Your question was clearly answered, but you are sitting there waiting for more and it does not come. It does not come because you are not specifically asking for a detailed intervention or assistance.

The wording of your questions and requests might also be so vague and ambiguous that the guides cannot respond clearly to you. Statements or directives such as, "I want to be healed," will often lead to disappointment. First of all, in this example, the word "want" will never send out a signal of receiving. It is truly the opposite of receiving. Another example might be, "Come and help me." Your guides can determine all types of different actions to take. Whatever the guides do, however, may not be anything you were hoping for. Yet at the same time, the guides might sense that they did indeed help you. I hope this makes sense to you.

Common words to avoid when communicating with the non-physical are:

- I want . . .

- I need . . .

- Help me . . .

- I hope for . . .

- Will you . . .

- Can I . . .

- Can you . . .

To get the sense and feel of these brief, ineffective phrases, place an ending on each one to make a complete statement. Now say each of them aloud or in your mind as if you are really requesting each one. For example, "Can I expect my grandmother to heal?" You might even get a yes, but in fact, the strongest energy of that question has very little to do with your grandmother. To the guides those particular words might vibrate more strongly of "Can I expect?" Another example might be, "I hope for a million dollars." The word "hope" does not send out a vibration of getting or receiving. One more example could be, "I want my body to heal." Can you sense the lack of direct clarity of each one of these particular examples?

Here is a portion of a session that describes someone feeling blocked and not clear in how to reach out to guides.

Client: I feel I have a block somewhere when I think about calling out to the sacred guides. I am sabotaging myself or I do not know how to do it. I feel like a little bud is inside my heart, and it begins to fill up as I call in my divine and sacred guides, but I cut it short, and I do not get anything in my mind. It is just a little feeling in my heart.

TZ: Tell me exactly what you "cut short." I want you to analyze that right now.

Client: I call on divine and sacred healing guides to heal my body when I sleep, to cleanse my body, to heal every cell, to restore my body, and build my immune system. But then I end up tuning out and I block it and lose track. I think it is because I really do not know how to call out to them for healing, so I wander off. My mind wanders. I do not finish it because it is too hard.

TZ: Your only effort should be to create the precise words in your commands. Commands are not being bossy. It is putting meaning behind your words. You just now stated the most beautiful command. I want you to write it down exactly as you said it a minute ago. Our only effort is to use the best and most precise words to our guides.

You and I could sit here and say, "Oh, help Susie," or you might call out and say, "Joe needs help now." Do you see how vague that is? Our thoughts are electrical. It is telepathy bouncing back and forth between our guides and us. If we put out a vague request, we get vague back. If we put out words and do not feel powerfully about it, then our words are just empty words. Write them out.

Client: So, I do not try to force anything with it?

TZ: Exactly. You only need to make sure you know who you are stating these words to. I always want the divine, sacred, and if holy feels right to you then use that word as well.

Client: So, make it specific and tailored to what you want, and go to the highest source for this and the right specialist and not any old body. That is just awesome. When I go to a specialist here (in the physical world) for my health I always say I want the best of the best but when I go to up there (points upward) I am not asking for the best of the best! Now I will get the best of the best of the guides. This makes so much sense to me.

Notice these next examples of using key words to send out concise, succinct verbiage:

"Tell me or show me now the exact point in my body that needs healing."

"Tell me or show me now the first step to take to release anger from my liver."

"What is the most perfect way to assist my grandmother now?"

"Tell me or show me the steps to receive financial abundance in my life now."

Ineffective statements are also caused by using too many words in one statement. Notice the examples above. They are succinct and to the point. There is no rambling. Do not create commands using two or more sentences. The more words you use, the more the meaning is clouded. The Universe receives a more well-defined signal from you when your question or request is in one brief sentence containing distinct words.

Now ask yourself these two questions and honestly sense the truthful answer. Do I ever pray against something to happen? Do I ever pray that something negative happens?

Here is a clear example of praying against something. A self-employed professional kept having two things consistently happen in his work. He consistently had many cancellations or people just not showing up for the appointments. He shared with me that he was praying all the time about his business struggles. When I asked what words he was using in his prayers, he said, "Dear God, please stop all the cancellations and no-shows from happening to me."

Can you see that he was praying against something happening and he was also using the exact words in his prayers that he did not want? After recognizing that he was praying against something, he changed the words within the prayer. Two things about this example:

1. A prayer is just like a command.

2. Never use the words in a prayer that you are trying to stop or get rid of. In this man's example, he was using the words "cancellations" and "no-shows". Those two words had the strongest vibrations because of his emotions about them. So, the strongest signal he was sending out was cancellations and no-shows. The Universe is neutral about what we ask for, so it kept giving him exactly what he asked for and exactly what he was praying against.

3. Carefully create the prayer using the most positive words. He easily changed his prayer to: "God, constantly and consistently fill all my weekly appointments with people who need my services and appreciate my services. Amen." Guess what happened? Within a week his business blossomed with people who were excited to see him and deeply appreciated his efforts for them.

Manifesting anything in your life is based on clear and distinct words, commanding it with feelings, but it is also about your expectations. Manifesting in your life will only take as long as you think it will take. If you think something will take months to happen, then that thought energy sends out a signal of slowness to not allow your request to happen until months go by. What you manifest depends on:

• Your correct usage of detailed words.

• Your positive, powerful feelings of commanding.

• Your expectations of how long something will take to happen.

Stop Now and Notice Yourself with Fascination

Notice yourself as you consider the key points we just discussed. What words have you been using? Are you clearly receiving from the old words you are accustomed to praying or commanding? What specific ways and words will empower your efforts?

Is it Okay to Command Spirits and the Universe?

In the past, I constantly used beautiful affirmations to speak, request, or even beg my guides to help with this or that. I rarely noticed a difference. Then I remembered that twenty years ago I studied the teachings of St. Germain. The word "command" kept being used. I thought . . . Command! What on earth are they talking about to command spirit! It was alarming to me. And now, all these decades later, it is not alarming to me, but it might be alarming to you.

Computers need commands to work for you. Spirit also needs commands to work with you and function for you. Let's examine the meaning of the word "command". To command the Universe, to me, signifies a very clear order or statement. To have a clear order, one must use very clear wording and really mean exactly what you say. It is not about being the boss or even becoming bossy or overbearing. But it does signify feeling the importance of what you are declaring in an intense way.

When you speak to your guides or ask questions, you must use precise, detailed words, and you must mean it when you say it. Every thought we think is an electrical burst out to the Universe. It is real. So, make it clear and truly have feelings and conviction when you interact with the Universe. Be a powerful link in the structure of the cosmos.

This mentoring client is trying to find out why her commands are not working well.

Client: I am struggling to receive intuitive information. When I checked just now, it's like everything is coming together and it is all sticking together like mush.

TZ: Now take the first thing that pops into your awareness when I ask you this. Where is all the mush located right now?

Client: The mush all comes together right here. (She points to her forehead.) I cannot think or concentrate. It is like a cloud there and it is not letting me have joy. I think sadness, and I cannot put a smile on my face. Since all of that, there are times that I cannot see through the cloud. It is trying to block me from doing my healing work.

TZ: I want you to ask your guides, "Why is it there and why do you keep getting interfered with even as you do your commands for protection?"

Client: I am told that I do not believe that I am really powerful, and I do not feel strong as I do the commands. So, the words are not sending out a powerful signal. It is a weak signal.

TZ: So, there is a bit of you that still does not recognize your own power. You still do not recognize that you are a powerhouse. I have goosebumps. You do not believe that you are more powerful than the negative entities. You do not believe that you are more powerful than the living people who are against you. You are always leaving yourself vulnerable because you have a belief that you are not powerful. That belief weakens your energy field.

Client: I looked within my abdomen and there was death and heaviness. I get a feeling of fear and anxiety, and it goes up to my throat.

TZ: Let's both ask the fear where it is coming from? (Long pause.)

Client: I could hear the word death and a banana skin. But I could not see anything.

TZ: Okay, what I just did was command, "Show me or tell me now the exact point of origin causing Jane's fear of her power." Now when I said that, I received two different points in time. In your current life as a child. I get five years old and eight years old.

There were multiple times when you were emotionally and maybe physically pushed and abused and beaten down. They did this to tell you that they are in control and not the kid in you. Does that make any sense to you?

Client: Well, funny you say that. When I grew up I had a sense that some form of abuse took place. My dad was always shouting and arguing at my mother, and I was always in the middle, and I do not know how I got there. I always had a fear when he went out drinking, and I would go into fear when he came home.

TZ: I do not see physical abuse, but you were constantly pushed down. That is emotional abuse. What you may not be remembering is two things. I see your dad yelling and telling you that you are just a kid and to stay out of it. He kept pushing and pushing you down. You were in the middle all the time, but you were never able to stop their fighting. Were you ever able to stop them? You could not ever resolve the situation and get them to change. This inability to make any change has carried over into your adult life, and now you continue to feel powerless over anything negative. You keep getting interfered with by negativity. You have been left vulnerable. You now think that negative dead people and negative nonhuman beings are more powerful than you are. You are clearly, clearly more powerful than you know right now.

Client: Okay, I agree with that.

TZ: Do you see now that this is getting in the way of you being a powerful healer for yourself and for others?

Client: Yes, I see that.

TZ: This is so big and important that my guides are saying this is the primary purpose for your current life. It is for you to realize your strength and power and the healer in you. Now here is the second thing I picked up.

I am shown a past life where you were the healer of the village. Someone died in the village of high importance. You were the healer, so you were punished. They tied huge stones on you and threw you in deep water. As you were sinking, you looked up at the sun.

Client: As you said that, I remembered that in this life when I was about seven, I was in a boat that tipped over, and I was rolling around the bottom of the sea and looking up at the sun. They grabbed me and pulled me up!

TZ: My guides are saying that you were given similar experience in this life that was repeating that experience in your past life. Again, it was a signal so you can heal those moments!

Client: Oh! I have goosebumps. I feel so really, really cold like I was then.

TZ: You were powerless in the past life and in your current life, so it is time for you to learn about this and heal it. You decided that you are powerless. And you are not powerless! This is big, and this is beautiful and profound information.

I not only have my personal experiences as an intuitive, but I also have the experiences and testimonials of tens of thousands of people who have read my books, taken my live or recorded courses, and have mentored with me on an individual basis. At this point of my experiences, not one single person has ever informed me that commanding has been negative in any way.

The Universe, our body, and our soul are electrically pulsing frequencies vibrating at different rates but vibrating all together within one extraordinary system. The Universe has structures in place that are often called Universal laws. To simply describe the structure of the Universe, our body and our soul is to describe it as electrically alive, pulsing frequencies vibrating at different rates but vibrating all together within one extraordinary system. We humans have so much choice that we have the choice to be power co-creators or weak creators within the system. That also means we humans have a choice to send and receive weak or powerful signals within the Universe.

Let's use those same examples of commands mentioned above:

- *Tell me or show me the exact point in my body that needs healing.*

- *Tell me or show me now the first step to take to release anger from my liver.*

- *What is the most perfect way to assist my grandmother now.*

- *Tell me or show me the steps to receive financial abundance in my life now.*

Just for practice, pick one of the commands that might be useful in your personal life. First just repeat it out loud or in your mind. Then repeat it and deeply mean it from your heart and soul . . . Now that is a command. Clear words with clear feelings.

Commanding is not about trying to be the boss. Commanding is essentially sending out the clearest, most concise, most power-packed electrical frequency of thought along with the most arousing energy of feelings to empower each thought vibration. Commanding in this way straightforwardly sends out a signal that is undeniably rich with energy and clear with words.

Stop Now and Notice Yourself with Fascination

Notice now if it makes sense to command when you consider the true meaning of the word.

Send Clear Signals by Visualizing

Clear wording of our commands is the primary pathway to communicate with the non-physical realms. Visualizing is another important pathway as well. Picturing a scene or an event in your mind's eye by using your imagination is the same as sending out an advertisement on a billboard alongside a highway. Picturing an image in our mind and interweaving happy, delighted emotions is like turning on neon lights around the billboard. Positive visualization honestly creates an energetic symbol. Symbols tell a complete story in a single picture. Spirit recognizes that positive story as a clear command.

The key is to create the image in your mind exactly as you want it to be and to feel as if you already have it in your life. I will share one of my personal examples of the power of visualization. I knew I was going to move to a certain area in the near future. I began to create a clear image in my mind of the property outside of the city in a rural area. I wanted to have an open view of the sky because I used to live in New Mexico, and I needed the freedom that the sky gives me. I wanted a house on some acres of land that was private. That was important to me because I grew up on a farm and loved the outdoors as well.

I roamed around all day with a realtor but found nothing that fit those images at all. She had one more place to show me. She slowed down as we approached the driveway. I looked out and said, "This is it!" My realtor responded, "We are not even on the property and you haven't even seen the house yet." I said with delight, "That's true, but I am buying this place!" It had everything I asked for with my verbal commands to the universe, but also everything that I visualized in my mind's eye while creating feelings of happiness and success. Precise words with conviction and clear visualizations with positive feelings cast a distinct command to the non-physical realms.

Yes to Meditating and Yes to Listening

Many Christians have questioned meditation. They have been told that it might open themselves up to negative forces. This has caused a great deal of concerns for many people struggling to understand. They are told that they must pray, and the most important thing to do is to talk to God.

The topic of most prayers are focused toward beseeching, pleading, or hoping for something for ourselves and for our loved ones. But when I ask people if they pause and listen and receive the information, they all say, "No! That never occurred to me!"

Talking at someone, even if it is God, is only one half of good communication. When does listening and receiving enter into prayers with God? Meditation is a sacred, deeply prayerful time. Meditating is setting aside a few moments to listen and to receive. How could sitting in a quiet moment open us up to danger? Does that mean if we keep very busy and keep constantly talking, we are safer? That just does not make any sense to me. Meditation is special individual moments to give to ourselves. It is settling down to allow yourself to listen and finally receive some answers to your requests.

To be clear, meditation is not the only way to listen. Meditation is a way to train yourself to listen and to receive. But in truth, one of my goals for you is to communicate continually with your guides, the Universe, and with God. My hope for you is to have one foot in the physical and one foot in the non-physical at the exact same time. That is the true balance in life because you are both physical and non-physical at the same time.

There are two ways to focus your meditative times. One is to go into a quiet stillness of sensing without thinking. The other is to offer a focused thought or a focused question in a more contemplative, reflective manner, then sit in stillness, noticing and receiving information. Meditation is not about doing. It is about listening and receiving. Here are basic steps to accomplish either one of these meditative options:

Simple Steps to Meditate and Listen

1. Sit upright, not stiff, but physically comfortable:
   - Do not cross arms or legs, lower shoulders, feet flat on the floor, allow teeth to part and rest the jaw, let your tongue rest on the roof of your mouth. Balance your head on top of your spine. Feel the alignment.

2. Close your eyes and feel them in their resting place.

3. Notice your thoughts with no judgment at all:
   - Welcome each thought and then release it. Do not fight against your thoughts or try to get rid of them. Feel the flow of your thoughts. Let your thoughts come in and then release them. Release each thought as it comes in. Pleasantly repeat this: Notice and release, notice and release, notice and release.

4. Notice your breath. Notice, without any criticism, each time your thoughts return to feeling your breath.

5. Breathe in the following manner:

- Feel the breath move into your chest. Feel your breath flow all around your heart. Slowly breathe down into the depths of your abdomen. The muscles of your abdomen will move outward as you inhale, making room for your breath. Relax your abdomen as you exhale. If you wish, slowly count one and two as you inhale. Now exhale at a slightly longer count than you inhale. If you inhale at the count of two then exhale at the count of three, do not push your breath in any way. Only notice.

6. Notice that you inhale and pause for a split second and exhale and pause for a second. Do not make yourself pause. Only notice the pause in your natural rhythm. Inhale—pause—exhale—pause—inhale—pause. Now notice the stillness inside of each pause.

7. Your stillness is in the pause . . . Feel your Soul . . . It sounds different from your mind.

- Practice for 2–5 minutes only.

- Practice anywhere and everywhere.

Essential Points

- Commanding is not about trying to be the boss.

- Commanding sends a clear, concise, power-packed electrical frequency with the most arousing energy within your request or question.

- You must use precise words or nothing can happen. Guides can only respond at the same energetic level that you send to them.

- You must pause, listen, and notice images to receive responses.

- Precise words with conviction and clear, positive visualizations cast a distinct command to the non-physical realms.

- You can be a weak link or a powerful link in the system. It is your choice.
- Manifesting only takes as long as we think it will.

Chapter 10

Intuitively Communicate and Develop
a Relationship with Your Guides

"This woo-woo non-physical shit is real. It would be
foolish to act like it's not there. It is what rings true."
—Robert Toth

You are Never Alone but You Do Have Choices

Sometimes a client tells me that it does not feel correct for them
to work with guides because they think they should only work
directly with God. I respond to them with this thought: If you have
a large pothole in your street, do you call the president or prime
minister of your country or do you call the local number listed for
street repair? Do you go to the one in charge of everything or the
one in charge of potholes?

The Universe itself is an energetic system. Within this highly
complex system is also a system of ceaseless choices for you and
every human on the planet. One of your greatest choices in this life
is to work, or not to work, with the spirit of the Universe and your
guides. It is totally up to you. This system communicates with you
constantly . . . It is forever and it is ceaseless. It is also neutral about
what you do with your energy, your body, your actions, and they
are neutral about your decision to work with them as a team, or
not to.

Many times we leave our spirit guides, but our divine and
sacred guides never leave us. But they also will not push into your

life. I have noticed that it is more powerful to call spirit in daily. Daily commands are best because our entire existence revolves around the natural cycles of the earth. The earth revolves, seasons revolve, the moon revolves, you are revolving. We have days and nights that revolve over and over, and many things are happening during that 24-hour cycle. I encourage you to call them in every morning and then again at bedtime. I also communicate with them constantly throughout my day.

You might discover that you have different requests to your spirit helpers for your daytime hours and different requests for your sleep time. For example, I have specialty guides for my sleep time because there is so much more happening than just sleeping. Our sleep time is a specialty time in our 24-hour cycle. That part of our cycle needs and deserves distinct guides to oversee our activities.

Here is a detailed interaction with a client regarding calling out to divine guides, deceased people, and our ancestors. Notice her fears and worries and how she became alarmed about questioning spirits.

Client: I get information from deceased people and from other beings, but I am not sure how I know these things.

TZ: Do you know where the information is coming from?

Client: No. I have no idea. Nothing at all.

TZ: I want you to do three things. One: Get more in charge of what is happening. Two: Find out who is telling you the information and what level of information it is. Three: Ask more questions of the guides and anyone else who is showing up.

Would you now call out to a divine and sacred guide to come to you?

Client: What if he does not come?

TZ: The guides will come if you call out very specifically for a divine and sacred guide.

Client: (Long pause) I think someone is here. My body got warmer.

TZ: Now. When we talk to them, we must be very precise and ask very short questions. Then we must pause and take whatever jumps into our mind. So, your first question to ask might be: "Are you the guide who has been assisting me?"

Client: I get a "yes" because my body is rocking from front to back. Wow!

TZ: Okay, ask him this: "Is he a guide who has reached the level of divine and sacred?"

Client: I did not know that I can ask that! I think maybe I should not ask questions. I am not trusting myself or I'm afraid. I grew up in the church and always heard not to do these things . . . But I asked and the guide at first said no, and now a guide says yes.

But now I have guides here and I saw a sad little boy in my mind's eye and then later he came to my house and he is alive. And I have deceased people here too. It is a mess! I think I have no control! I am just here to help, and I have no control!

TZ: I want you to be more in charge of this and be more in control of it, and here is why: Spirits of people who have died are often very needy, and they will come to you constantly. If you do not get in charge of this, they will wear you out. I hope you will be okay when I help you be more in charge.

Client: That makes complete sense because this is a mess, and I do not know where you should even start? (Now we are both laughing.)

TZ: I hope you will be okay to be more in charge. Right now, you have guides coming in. Some say they are guides and some are deceased people coming in. Then you also see an alive child coming to you before the child even arrives physically in your home.

Let's begin by you telling me what type of guide you want first to help you? They have specialty areas. What area do you want?

Client: I feel like I would like to heal people the most. To find their light and to awaken and get out of the dark. I would like to be able to see into the person at a distance.

TZ: Let's put this in clear words and say it in your mind. You could say the following:

I call out to the universe. I request right now a divine and sacred guide who specializes in healing and bringing people to the light inside of them.

Client: That is just right.

TZ: Then go ahead and say these words out into the universe and really feel that you mean it and feel the power of it.

Client: (Long pause) I notice some positive energy.

TZ: Ask this guide if they are divine and to show themselves to you in your mind's eye.

Client: It is a man. I see only his face. He has dark hair and moustache and beard. Young.

TZ: Ask him more questions such as, "What do you need to do to work well with him for others?" One question at a time. You must ask the question and then wait. Take the first thing that leaps into your mind.

Client: He says we are already working together. He says his name is Jesus. But I cannot believe it. I do not deserve his presence. (Tearful) He is too elevated.

TZ: But you asked for a guide who is elevated. He came to you and that should tell you that you are deserving, and you deserve to work together.

Client: (Quiet and still crying) It is unbelievable.

TZ: Well, you now have Jesus, but you will also have many more guides who have different specialties. Jesus has come forward for me as well, but I have many guides along with him. For example, you also have so many dead people coming to you because you are a natural medium. You might have a specialty guide who will help group the dead people or ask them to line up and wait for you, so you are not so overwhelmed.

So, I want you to communicate more and ask more questions and give spirit people more directions. Even deceased people are still alive, and they have their thoughts. They will communicate. Give them directions because many are confused and need your help.

Client: I have also been calling in ancestors to help deceased people. I call them in because the dead person already knows their own ancestors, and this will help them.

TZ: But I want you to understand if you just call out to ancestors on behalf of someone else, you are not being clear and specific about who you want. Ancestors can be very negative and bad, and some are wonderful. Would you be okay to call out for the most loving and aware ancestors? That way you do not get the "bad guys," who are also within the ancestors.

Client: Oh! That makes so much sense. Do you know that no one, not even my husband, knows about these things that I see and do? You do not think I am crazy!

TZ: No, you are not crazy at all. You are very intuitive.

Now here is a mentoring client who works with her divine and sacred guides for self-healing:

"Hope you don't mind me sharing a story with you, as I know you like stories . . . While sitting in the front room, I felt the urge to come into my little room and sit in the corner chair. As I did this, I closed my eyes, and there in front of me stood a monk. He was dressed in a cream-coloured robe and a brown rope belt. I couldn't see his face only his clothing. He then knelt down in front of me and told me that we needed to do a healing. So I sat quietly and went with it. He said he wanted to go to the stomach area which was like an orange bucket and he wanted to pull these two black strings out. I watched him as he pulled and pulled. It felt as if it went on for a long time. Then he filled the hole with light and the hole closed. He then went up to my throat and it looked like a royal blue diamond that split in half. Inside this diamond was a little glow of shining light. He then filled that with more light and as he did this, I began to cough and cough. Then the coughing stopped. The light inside was really bright and the diamond closed. After this, I watched as he picked up what looked like a singing bowl. As he lifted the singing bowl, the noise from it was like vibrations of bubbles. I felt very strong and could hear the music as it was reaching above me. Then as soon as it had gotten to the top of me, he left. What a healing thought! It left me knackered for two days!"

Stop Now and Notice Yourself with Fascination

What do you think about the constant, ceaseless moments of choice that you have in this life? Please consider working with your teams of guides. They are waiting patiently for an invitation. You must telepathically talk to them, but be careful and be clear with the words you use.

How to Call Your Specialty Guides—Be Careful and Be Clear!

Oh my goodness! People get into more trouble, trauma, and crises while calling out to guides than anything else I can think of at the moment.

- Remember how important each word is as you create thoughts within your brain?
- Remember that each thought, each phrase, each sentence rockets out into the world, then much farther out into the Universe?
- Remember that the spirit realms and the Universe must respond with the same energy that you put out to them?
- Remember that the highest energy creates the highest response?

- Remember you can be a weak link or a powerful link in the system? It is your choice.

This client talks to her guides about their skills.

TZ: When I ask you this question, what actually pops up? What is the struggle for you regarding working with your guides?

Client: Well, when I ask my guides a question, I can recognize a good six or eight guides that are there for different things. But should I have a clear picture in my head of what they look like, who it is, what their name is? How much detail should I have about them as I ask a question?

TZ: No. At least start with calling out for a divine and sacred specialist in something you want or need. Then really get to know them before you ask them questions. I do not take the time to bother to see them when I am actually working on myself or other people because I have already met them and have interacted with each one on my teams (before we begin to work together).

It is like my four professors who help me with teaching my courses and help me with the private mentoring sessions like we are doing right now. I do not see them or what they look like, but I can feel them and their divinity.

Client: That helps. I have a guide who really does not talk but takes me by the hand and says, "Look here first." Yet, I have another guide who is like a professor who gives me that information.

TZ: I think you are telling me that the guide who does not really talk is more like a specialist in pointing you in the right direction. Who shows you where the problem is. Ask her if that is her specialty, and she will answer you.

Client: Yes, she quickly says, "Go here first. Look here first. This is where you need to go." It's like a guy with a big flashlight zooming in."

TZ: Ask your laser beam guide if she is also supposed to give you information as well as where to look.

Client: She will show me where to look, but the information is coming from someone else.

TZ: See . . . you have a specialist to point to the exact location, and she is telling you that you have specialists for receiving more information and also specialists for healing.

All of these guidelines listed above especially apply when calling out and inviting guides into your life. Guides, like people, come in all levels of awareness and all levels of development just like us. Many times I am working with a client and their guides come forward and I see them. Occasionally, I see a guide standing back behind others. When I ask who that is and why they stand back behind others, I am often told that they are a student who is only to observe. That seems reasonable to me.

After a great deal of investigating, I have discovered that pretty much any dead person can offer to be a guide whether they have achieved that higher level of awareness or not. Dead people are mostly just dead people and have not achieved that level of insight, but think they can help out anyway. I have also witnessed deceased drug addicts, grandmas, great aunts, and old friends who state they are guides for my living client sitting in front of me. If you ask them if they have reached the blessed divine level they will tell you no and fade away.

Personally, I want the most mature, advanced celestial guides possible. I want the most evolved and the most sanctified guide possible. I will not accept anyone lower to guide me. Here is what it takes to receive that enhanced intensity of advancement in a guide:

- You must be meticulous when creating your commands to the Universe.
- You must use well-defined words that are exceptionally clear and distinct.
- These words must rule out any spirit thinking or wishing

that they could ride along with you or cling to your body and life.

This might surprise you, but there are words that seem good but, in fact, these words send out an energy signal that is blurred and too general.

The words never to use are: The best . . . The greatest . . . The highest . . . The supreme . . .

I ask people to never use these words when calling out for a guide for one reason. The negative and dark realms also have beings that are: The "best," the "greatest," the "highest," the "supreme," and the "revered."

Does this make sense to you? Many people are fooled and deceived when they call out for guides using these words. They unknowingly use these nebulous words which open their energy field and bodies to a full spectrum of negativity. That spectrum may include simple, opportunistic, negative deceased people all the way to the most negative entities possible and everything in between. The negative realm is real, it is complicated, and it can be hazardous. These negative entities can be removed and escorted to the Light, but it takes some effort to do so. People are usually terribly interfered with before realizing what has happened to them. (The exact steps to handle negativity are later in this book.)

I searched to find words with potent, forceful positive vibrations that cannot be confused with the negative aspects of the Universe. Notice the energetic feel of these words as you read them:

Divine . . . Sacred . . . Blessed . . . Sanctified . . . Hallowed . . . Pure . . . Holy . . .

The next step in calling out to the Universe for a guide is to define what type of guide you are asking for. Are you looking for health, abundance, better relationships, a great job, great communication, release of negative patterns, or something else? What words best describe what you need help with? I want a guide who meets the criteria in the words above, but I also want a guide who specializes in the area of life that I need help with. The earthly world has specialists in nearly every area of life. Plumbers and electricians usually specialize in commercial or residential buildings. Physicians and nurses specialize in specific areas of medicine. Lawyers specialize in estate planning or divorce or a multitude of other areas of law. Truck drivers need certain licenses.

I want a guide who meets the divine and sacred requirements and who is also a specialist in a specific area that I need assistance in. For example, people who attend my workshops often come up to me at breaktime. They are so delighted to tell me they see four columns of light standing behind me. I tell them that those are my four specialty guides who call themselves The Professors. They assist me to teach and present spiritual information during my courses. To receive guidance at that level of wisdom and clear honesty, I used this command:

I request divine and sacred guides who specialize in teaching spiritual wisdom to groups eager to learn, come work with me now.

Another example that I have used to assist me in writing all my books is this:

I call out to the divine and sacred guides who specialize in creating and writing books to teach others about the spirit world, come work with me now.

The two steps I am describing here are to:

1. Use fine and high vibrating words such as "divine," "sacred," "blessed," "sanctified," "hallowed," "holy," or "pure," to send the clearest signal that you only want the best of the best. No one else can get near to this level that you are requesting.

2. You want to command that only a specialist in the area you want assistance in can come near you. No one else can appear but one who excels in a specific field.

Basically, you have sent out a distinct, well-defined billboard shining in neon, glistening light out into the Universe, describing a narrow classification and quality of guide that you want. From now on, do not just call out to the Universe for help. Please take care to use your words wisely. You are powerful and your words are powerful. But it is up to you to function in the bright light of infinite love and to work only with guides who vibrate in that same light.

The next thought you might have is, "What kind of specialists are there to work with?" It seems to me that there is no end to the specialists. I have specialists and teams of specialists. I have teams for medical intuition. Each one on the team might be considered a sub-specialist. I have one who specializes in diagnosing, one excels in the heart, and so on. I have specialists for issues and topics such as relationships, marketing and promoting, communication, teaching workshops, and another for writing books. There are specialists for health and healing, for animal communication and care, specialists for computer issues, etc.

There are also special assignment teams for short-term projects. I do not worry or try to discern who comes forward in the team because they work out which individual steps up to do the task. There seems to be no end to the assistance that can be there for us. What is vitally important to remember is the quality of the guide. You want the divine and sacred, and you want a specialist.

Stop Now and Notice Yourself with Fascination

First, remember that working with the non-physical world will always, always seem like your imagination. Start by deciding what specialty area you want or need a specialist for. I would suggest a place to begin . . . Call out for a divine and sacred guide who specializes in working with you to receive accurate intuitive information.

What direction does the guide come from? Where does the guide stand when they arrive? Then notice the details of who arrives to assist you. What do they look like, feel like? Notice everything.

Don't Just Talk . . . Listen and Receive

You have just reached out and made contact with an extraordinary, elevated spirit guide specialist. Now what do you do? I want you to develop a relationship with this guide. I want you to use telepathy to communicate. Again, telepathy is our ability to send electrical pulses of thought back and forth from you to another and back again. What questions do you have for your specialist? Be curious. Who has arrived for you? Allow yourself to actually interview your guide to get to know them. Create an ongoing relationship with this guide and a deeper connection with each and every guide.

We humans tend to talk a lot to our guides and our deceased loved ones. We talk by having thoughts in our head, by praying, by directly commanding within our heads or out loud. But while teaching tens of thousands of people over the decades, I quickly discovered that the primary issue we humans consistently have is listening and receiving the information. How can that be?

I first learned, from a dead person, that living people do not listen. Through telepathy, he told me that he talks and talks and responds to this alive person all the time. The alive person was a client sitting in my office at the time. Her deceased loved one showed up as she was describing to me that she talks all the time to the deceased family member, but she never gets anything back from him. I could see him standing next to her, listening. He looked at me and projected this thought to me. "I answer her but she never listens."

We alive humans are not listening to our deceased loved ones, but we are also not listening to our guides. What is getting in the way? First, people really do not expect to get any answers from the dead or from the heavens. Second, when people do notice a thought jumping into their heads that might have come from a dead person, they immediately blow it off as their imagination and then immediately forget about it. Third, many people do not feel that they deserve to receive help from guides or even deserve to hear from the dead.

What chance do the dead or heavenly guides have to get through to us!

You are not bothering your dead people or your guides. The entire Universe is developing and expanding. We humans are not the only beings advancing. Guides are also developing as well. The deceased are continuing to learn too. It never stops. The more we work and interact with the guides, the more the guides achieve as well.

Do not paraphrase what spirit says to you. They are very literal and exact, so receive it without altering it. Do not assume something and do not wonder about what they just meant. Always, always, always ask more precise questions to get more precise answers and guidance.

Remember, intuitive communication is an ongoing dialogue and not just one question. Dialogue back and forth like you do with other living people. You talk . . . they listen . . . then they talk . . . and you listen and receive the pop.

Here are some examples of questions you might begin with. You think you will remember everything, but write down your interactions. You will have many guides to get to know and to work with.

Begin to dialogue with one guide at a time. Ask the questions one at a time. Listen and receive the answers popping into your mind:

- What name can I call you?
- How do you qualify as a specialist in ____?
- How will you help me with this issue?
- What should I look for when you contact me?
- How will I know that you are there?
- What is the first step I should take?
- How often can I call out to you?
- Why do I keep having this same type of problem?

Stop Now and Notice Yourself with Fascination

Our guides will always show up, and they will always respond in some way . . . either vague or specific since that is up to you. Did you allow yourself to receive the information? Did you discount it or minimize it or fail to trust what you received?
If you did any of those things . . . Stop it now. You are the only one who can open yourself up to the wisdom that is there for you.

Constant Protection Day and Night

Remember earlier in this book, I discuss how we are not meant to be encapsulated by crystal eggs or walls or any other type of boundary around us. Your greatest protection is the brightest light of your toroidal field shining from inside your entire body and glowing outward through every inch of your skin. Your natural toroidal is the best protection of all. I want you to feel invincible because of your glowing brightness.

Our guides are there to support our positive power too. It is a team effort. There are specialty guides for protection and empowerment. Archangel Michael is the most recognized as the protector and leader of an army of angels against the forces of evil. He is often depicted with a blue flaming sword. There are also a myriad of other entities who are considered protectors as well.

Call in and work with protection each day to continually build a constant protective field. Again, I ask that you take care in the wording of your commands for protection. Consider using one command during the day and another during your sleep time. During the day we are busy with the material world with material type struggles and issues. We humans are also very active during our sleep time, but we are active in different ways while we sleep. I personally love this command but it is only one of many.

> *My heart is a sacred space.*
> *My head is a sacred space.*
> *My body is a sacred space.*

My energy field is a sacred space.
My higher self is a sacred space.
My soul is a sacred space.

Some of our sleep time is spent with our brain firing off images and thoughts that have happened during the daytime. Our brain and subconscious is trying to sort out and process our work, our play, relationships, stresses, arguments, interactions with others, and so on. Spirit guides and also deceased loved ones come to us to talk things over. We astral project into other realms to learn or interact with others. We also astral project all throughout the earth plane as well.

Many people tell me that I come to them in their dreams. I myself remember many dreams where I just taught a class in India or in Germany or some other location. I remember dreams where I meet with my guides to learn something. I have also traveled into the astral plane where emotions and actions are raw and ugly. I awake knowing I was trying to learn something or trying to save someone.

During the freedom of our sleep, without meaning to, we might place ourselves at risk because of being more vulnerable. Call out for a guide to work with you for protection.
An example of this command is:

The most divine and sacred guardian, come to me, (full name), now. Protect my physical body, my energy field, my spirit, and my soul at all levels and in all dimensions now.

Get to know your protector and dialogue with this guide. Find out exactly what the guide is doing to keep you safe. After creating a relationship with the protection guide, instruct them with a clear command such as these two examples:

My most holy and sacred Warriors of the Light . . . Completely and permanently remove all negativity from my body, mind, and energy field now. Keep all negativity away from me and keep me away from all negativity. So be it!

This is another example to use for your safety but also to remove any negative interference you might already be aware of.

I request the divine and sacred Protector to collect and totally extract all negative entities, all negative cords, all negative connections from my body, from my energy field, from my soul, and from my environment. Take it all now to the highest place for its transformation into Light and Love.

Constant Truths About the Spirit World

1. You are a spirit right now.
2. You are a spirit with other spirits right now.
3. You are not separate from the spirit world because you are constantly a part of it.
4. Guides want and need an invitation or request to participate in your life.
5. You are in charge of the invitation and what you request.
6. You must communicate with exceptionally clear words because spirits are exceptionally literal.
7. Guides have specialty areas and skills just like humans do.
8. They will respond to you in all kinds of unexpected ways.
9. Their messages are extremely subtle and come through many pathways.
10. Just like humans, guides love your gratitude too.

Essential Points

- You have constant and ceaseless moments of choice in this life.
- One of your greatest choices in this life is to work, or not to work, with the spirit of the Universe and your guides.

- You must be meticulous when creating your commands to the Universe.

- In a command, there are words to always use and words to never use.

- Allow yourself to receive wisdom from the universe. Everyone deserves to receive wisdom.

- Intuitive communication is an ongoing dialogue and not just one question.

- Your greatest protection is your toroidal field and your divine guide of protection.

- Placing an energetic barrier around you will block your ability to receive the positive.

Chapter 11

Intuitively Communicate with Deceased People—It's Not Too Late to Heal

"It is time to be the medicine, the uplifting music, the lamp in the darkness. Burst out with love. Be a carrier of hope. If there is a funeral, send them off with a song."

—Jack Kornfield

Death is Not the Enemy—Let's Talk About It

Yes. It's okay to talk about death. This is an extremely important section of this book because this will take your personal healing into a profound and meaningful depth.

Deceased people are everywhere. Spirit people are in and out of your house, your car, your work. They are in the grocery stores, the theatres, restaurants, and they are at your vacation spots. There is no place on this earth where people in spirit are not there. If you can adjust your mind to the fact that you are only one of billions of other spirits and some have physical bodies and some do not, then you are on your way to natural interdimensional experiences without fear.

When we leave our body, it is not the end. It is, however, an end for those who are left behind. We are often left with burdens of sorrow, regrets, memories of all types, burdens of responsibility, and so on. Healing is needed for living and the deceased. It is not too late to heal the dead, the dying, the living, and as a result to heal ourselves. Living people who are now preparing to make their transition into death do not think it is too late to heal. People who are now deceased come to me nearly every day, and even they do not think it is too late to heal.

Hear me . . . My goal is to remove your fear of the dead right now. Your role as an intuitive will include being a medium which is a deeply natural part of your intuitive skills. As you read this book you are a person in spirit. That spirit is the aliveness inside of your body. Spirits are usually all around you even if you do not want to notice them. They come and go just as we come and go throughout our day. Dead people are still just real people, and they are still alive. When a person in spirit arrives, I simply treat them as a "surprise living person" who wants or needs something, and with the help from my guides I am here to assist them. Assisting the dead will always assist your own healing in new and sometimes surprising ways.

As you read this book, and especially now as you read this section, I want you to know that you can heal your painful relationships with people who have already died. Even though someone has died, it is not too late to heal the old issues and the old wrongs. It is not too late to heal traumatic events where the dead person was the wrongdoer. Healing can also be accomplished if you feel you failed the deceased in some way. Believe me when I say once again, it is not too late to heal yourself, the deceased, or the painful events and memories between both of you.

Many people in spirit will be your own family members, friends, or acquaintances. Just like the living, the dead have a lot to say about things, and they are here to finally say it. The dead, like the living, may be confused, angry, lost, or obsessed with something in the physical and often do not understand what is happening to them. Some of your deceased family or friends are eager to get a message to you. They often want to resolve an issue with you personally or with someone in the family. They might want to simply tell you how well they are doing now that they rose from their physical body. Remember you are a spirit with a body and they are a spirit without a body. That is the only difference and there is nothing to be afraid of. They may arrive unexpectedly, or you can call out to them and they will arrive with your request. This is a time for you to heal in an unexpected way.

One of my mentoring clients had an old rule embedded into her mind. It was placed there a long time ago. She described to me how she would see deceased people nearly every day in her home, but she absolutely refused to dialogue with all the dead people that kept showing up. She, in fact, always chased them out of her home on a daily basis, and I kept seeing them run to the neighbor's house just so they could remain close to her.

I asked this woman to understand two points:

1. Deceased people are still real people who need some type of assistance or they would not be coming to you.

2. Spirit people still have their own energy field and some level of their old personality. They are usually struggling or searching for something. The energy of a needy spirit person might directly interfere with your own health. So, as you assist the spirit person with their needs, you are keeping yourself healthier at the same time. Many times their primary need is assistance to cross over. More on that in chapter 23.

One day during our session, she had a breakthrough. She realized she was holding onto a very old rule given to her by her grandmother. Grandmother said, "You are to never speak to the dead." My client embedded that into her mind and absolutely refused to go against her grandmother's command. My client suddenly realized that this was her grandmother's rule and it no longer needed to be her rule. My client then realized that she is a skilled medium and apparently the dead know that as well.

Recognizing yourself as a natural medium and assisting spirit people who come to you is yet another pathway for your own healing. They do not have their physical body, but they still exist and are still alive, active, learning, and will interact with you if you accept them. They will respond to you, and you can respond to them. You can learn and advance together and no longer live in fear that a dead person might show up in the night.

The deceased might have already approached you to bring a healing between the two of you. Did you ignore them or decide that spirits do not exist and you just imagined it? Did you decide that you could not possibly be picking up thoughts from the dead? I will repeat this again: we humans are a powerful link in the healing system of the universe. You can communicate with the deceased as if you picked up the phone and called them. You can now work out your issues, completely and permanently heal yourself, and spark the same level of healing within the soul of the deceased.

It is important that you be in complete charge as you interact with spirit people. They will actually do exactly as you request, but you must be specific about your wants and needs as well. My house becomes so full of dead people that I often find myself commanding loudly inside my mind, "I am still in the physical and need my sleep. Everyone must be completely quiet now! I will meet you in the sunroom at ten a.m. tomorrow to assist you with your needs!" Just minutes prior to that command, the house had sounds of cracking wood in the walls, paper rustling downstairs, or dishes clunking in the kitchen. When all these unlikely sounds occur in your home they are only trying to get your attention. They are not trying to terrorize you. There is no need to be afraid because they will do exactly what you ask as long as you are clear and mean what you say to them.

While working with spirit people, you can continue on with a conversation for as long as you want. Please note, however, that if they have approached you or arrived at your home, they have a reason or a goal. I suggest you direct your dialogue to the issue they have. If you can help them by sharing their message with someone, then do that if possible. If it is not possible, tell them so and assist them in some other way.

Many of them have not crossed over into the Light. They do not cross over for many different reasons because they are different individuals. Some of the deceased will be people that you know and even love, and some are strangers. They will show up and you have no idea why they have come to you. Most of them will have no idea why they have arrived at your home either. They come to you because intuitives feel different and look different. Regardless, they need you in some way but they often cannot put it into words. Sometimes the deceased will explain dramatic reasons for approaching you:

- Obsessed with material property such as land, a house, furniture, etc.
- Obsessed with an alive individual.
- Feel they were too terrible in life and do not deserve to cross over.
- Trying to resolve old conflicts with certain people.
- Attempting to continue sensations and feelings that they had in life caused by things such as alcoholism, drugs, or sex.
- Many have no idea they died and have left their physical body.

Here is an excellent example of communicating with a negative spirit showing up in my client's kitchen one evening. Take note: No matter how ugly or sinister the dead person is, they arrived because they need help or need to communicate.

Client: We were at the dinner table and I got that feeling. I had the feeling that I have some work to do. So, I had the feeling that this is a guy that I did not want to hang around here. This was the first one that gave me the creeps. I also had such a headache.

TZ: Yes, some of them will.

Client: Not in a way that scared me, but I had the sense that this one was negative and creepy and there was something not right about this one (spirit person). This was the first one I interacted with that was creepy. It was not good for him to allow him to hang around here.

TZ: Well, this was more about how it is not good at all for you or your boyfriend to have him around you. So, what were your next steps with the creepy guy?

Client: I sat down even though I had a migraine that night; I sat down to help him. I heard his name. I asked him, "Are you aware you are dead?" He did, in fact, know that. I asked him, did he know that being here is not helping him in his own progression? He said he was not aware of that. I could sense that there was something about his face and it was creepy. I engaged him and told him that I am an expert for people like him, and I will help him now. I told him I called in specialty guides who will help him, and I asked him to count how many came for him. There were three. I told him to feel the love that they had for him. I had to wait a while. (She was waiting for the specialty guides to follow her commands and take him to the Light for his transformation.)

TZ: Earlier, you told me that you do not see anything, but you keep mentioning his face. I think that you are seeing. You are truly seeing spirit and not realizing it.

Client: I think that if I am seeing things, I must see it the way I am seeing you right now. I don't do that. I just see things in my imagination, and that does not count!

TZ: Oh my goodness sakes! Seeing with your eyes open like you are seeing me and seeing with your eyes closed are two different pathways of receiving clairvoyance. Both will always feel like your imagination, but both are real.

Client: Really, Tina? I just thought, I don't see things like Tina does. I do not see dead people just walk up to me and I see them. It always happens when my eyes are closed. It's all in my imagination.

TZ: No, it's not. It will always feel like imagination. I want you to stop saying, "It was my imagination," because your eyes were closed. No, eyes open or eyes closed are both pathways to receive clairvoyance. Make that adjustment right now.

Client: I have been saying that because I do not think I am that evolved, not that developed, I'm not that gifted because I do not see with my eyeballs open.

TZ: One of the main reasons we tend to see more with our eyes closed is that they have to be pretty dense and more physical. If they are that dense they either just recently left their physical body and have not crossed over or they were very negative. Negative deceased people who lived in negative ways tend to have more density, more thickness or stickiness because negativity has more density to it.

You have been pointing at the right side of your head. Was there something wrong with the right side of this man's face?

Client: Yes, it was so vivid to me that the right side part of his face was drippy like his skin was melting off. I got a feeling about him and his life and his nasty look. It was not good. But it was the first time that I felt I was really seeing something.

TZ: You have been pointing at the right side of your head and you earlier said you were getting a migraine. Was your headache on that same side?

Client: Yes!

TZ: I want you to see that it was not your headache. You were getting an energetic signal from the nasty spirit person about the damage he had to his head. You were not getting anything from him, but you were getting the signal about it. I am right now getting that he had the right side of his head blown off by a gun.

Client: That seems exactly right. Now I realize that.

TZ: Remember when we are getting signals, and especially signals of pain, do this command: *I recognize that signal. It is not mine. Out of me now.* Then you actually push it out of you because it is not yours to have.

One of my mentoring clients was meeting with me to build her intuitive abilities. We were meeting virtually so I could see the room in her home behind her. As our session went on, I kept noticing a deceased person standing in the corner of her room. We were focusing on medical intuition for others, so I did not mention it until the end of our session. I informed the client that intuition does include mediumship, the ability to interact with dead people. I told my client that I had been perceiving a spirit person behind her during our session today. Instead of me telling her what he looks like and other information I was picking up from him, I asked her to check in to practice connecting with the deceased. She checked and said the following:

"This was interesting. I felt the deceased person was a male friend who passed away about three weeks ago. Our families had been close friends, and I heard that he wanted me to make sure they were going to be okay. He wants me to help them adjust to his passing. He says he chose me because I was a 'bright light.' At his funeral, I had a conversation with a man there that I hadn't seen for years. I also felt he (the deceased) wanted me to reconnect with that man (living man at the funeral home) so that I might be able to have a loving relationship similar to what the deceased had experienced with his first wife and second life partner. After he communicated (this information) with me, I could see two guides walking him into a light-filled hallway to cross over. This is certainly not what I expected to get, but that's the 'pop' that came. Wow!"

My client was amazed with the interaction she just had with the male spirit standing behind her.

Spirit People Communicate in Different Ways

A week before her birthday, my sister called to tell me that she was feeling our mother so strongly, and so she was talking to Mother more and more. The feeling of our mother was getting stronger every day with my sister. Then the day before my sister's birthday she called me again. She said, "I have something to tell you and show you." I said, "Great," but she sounded so strange I was a bit worried. She held up a very old photo of the lake cottage that our grandparents used to own and said, "Have you ever seen this photo?" I saw an ancient printed photo of the cottage with our parents sitting on the front porch. Then I said, "Wow, where did you get that? I have never seen that photo before." My sister described how she had never seen it before either. Then she went on to say that the old photo was laying on her dresser in the bedroom when she got up this morning. Clearly our mother was attempting to get my sister's attention and send a type of communication in the form of an ancient photo.

A professional medical intuitive shared her story of her father being stuck in fear of the unknown heavens.

"It was a cold day in January when a routine checkup with my dad's oncologist for his rare blood disease suddenly turned gray. He had been battling critically low platelet counts and had received several blood transfusions for over ten years, and his oncologist never thought it would turn to leukemia but it did. I will never forget the energy and the news she carried with her when she walked into the room and delivered the news that his blood work had indicated that my dad had full-blown leukemia and only had six months to live. It was like a lightning bolt had struck and shocked our family to its core. My dad, mom, and I sat there in disbelief as my dad was scrambling for the answers and the realization of the chapters of his life suddenly coming to an end.

"My family's spiritual upbringing was deeply rooted in Baptist principles and philosophies, and since I was a little girl I had personally experienced angels and loving spirits interacting with my family on a day-to-day basis. But as I got older and continued to attend Sunday School and church I was told that 'spirits' were not necessarily a good thing. This perspective really challenged what I was seeing and experiencing, and then as I got older and started studying and researching the metaphysical and shamanic realms on my own, I realized that this is as vital and important as my Baptist upbringing, and I began blending and melding the two into my own spiritual walk.

"That day in the doctor's office when we received my dad's prognosis, I noticed there were new angels and guardians surrounding us, along with other family members that had made their transitions. It's as if they were offering their assistance, love, and support for the months ahead, and I was hoping that my mom and dad could see and feel their love and comfort as much as I could that day.

"As far as the spiritual spectrum, my dad wasn't one to open up and talk about his feelings and emotions and especially talking about God and the Bible, but he began opening up and asking questions about heaven and what happens after we die. We all knew the Bible's interpretations of heaven and the afterlife, but when my dad started to really wonder it's as if it created an opening for me to share the metaphysical and shamanic realms with him.

"We had several insightful conversations around the biblical sense of heaven in relation to the essence of the soul and what happens after we die, and I noticed after several of these conversations that my father's spirit began to gently shift and explore the outer realms of his physical body. I could see in his eyes when he would be fully engaged in relation to being half here and half 'there'.

"And it was within a few weeks of my dad exploring the outer spiritual realms that he finally decided to gently take his last breath and make his transition to heaven, or at least we thought he did. And this is when it became very interesting . . . My personal faith and belief systems were challenged, but the practices of Tina's medical intuition workshop about working with specialist guides came full circle.

"Several months after my dad had passed, I was driving along the interstate, and he suddenly dropped in from 'heaven' and appeared in the passenger seat of my car. He was in a tizzy, full of fear and angst and talking a hundred words a minute about 'heaven' not being like the 'heaven' that was described in the Bible and how the pastors talked about it in church at the pulpit and ranting that he didn't trust what he was seeing and being asked to enter into the next stage of his life. He was rambling on about all of our spiritual conversations we had and was frantically asking for my help and needing validation that what he was experiencing was safe and okay to enter into.

"And I immediately thought of Tina's protocol of calling in the angels, specialist guides, and loved ones to surround my dad with so much love, comfort, and light in helping calm his fears, embrace the light, and allow him to fully make his transition. It was in that moment that I witnessed my dad being surrounded and loved by his mom, dad, stepdad, brother, and so many other loved ones along with the angels and guides. I called out to him, and I promised I would take care of Mom and ensured him that it was his time to go and be free. I shared and expressed how loved he is and how safe it was for him to go with the angels, guides, and loved ones. He proceeded to slowly walk with his angels, then he paused for a moment and gently looked over his left shoulder and told me how much he loved me and thanked me for helping him. He told me how proud he was of me for embracing my spiritual walk and sharing it with him. It was one of the most beautiful healing moments I have seen, and I am so grateful to have witnessed his angels, guides, and family members taking him to 'heaven'."

Later on, after sharing her experience with her father, Beth shared this with me.

"It's an interesting journey, and Tina, I keep hearing you say: 'You can't make this up.' My Baptist upbringing boxed me in for so many years until I was in college and started to explore different religions and realized I have to create my own spiritual walk and pave my own path to what feels right for me.

"Just so you know, you and your teachings have helped me feel like I am not crazy for the things I have witnessed, seen, and experienced. I will never forget when I took your workshop for the first time in Chicago and I was sitting there with my mouth wide open when you were sharing the advanced information on the third day. I was like, 'Holy shit—there is actually somebody else who has experienced some of the same craziness that I have! And I truly thought I was the only one that had ever seen the broad spectrum of light to dark. And then when you brought forward the techniques on how to work with these energies, it all clicked and started making sense and I felt so empowered."

Steps to Telepathically Communicate with the Deceased

You can talk back and forth just as if they are real because they are real. Send them telepathic questions through your thinking mind. Imagine someone calling you on the phone needing to talk:

1. Feel and know the powerful energy of your own thoughts. They are electrical vibrations extending outward to the person in spirit.

2. Begin by asking the deceased person to tell you their name.

3. Pause to receive the response.

4. Notice the instant pop of telepathic information into your mind. It will come as instant words, sentences, or pictures.

5. Respond to them with your own telepathic thoughts. Keep sentences short and to the point.

6. Create a back-and-forth dialogue to discover what they want or need.

7. Notice if they feel positive, negative, distraught, afraid or confused.

8. Be clear and be in charge. Learn together and heal together.

Here is a brief excerpt from a session where my client realizes how she is powerfully assisting deceased people to cross over.

Client: Oh! My goodness, I want to talk to you about this. Ever since class (Become a Medical Intuitive Workshop) I have had so much work and so much has happened. One or two times a week I have a lot of dead people showing up and I have been helping them move up and out. That has been the best and biggest thing that has happened since class. I'll get an intuitive feeling and I will know that someone is around. I power up and I start engaging and I quickly learn that there is someone there. Then I think . . . did I just do that? Did I just help someone? It made me feel so good to help someone. Is word out on the street that they know I can help? I have never felt scared because of your training, and I always feel confident. I feel they need help, and they are just a client. I am very happy to be able to help them. I follow the steps strictly and clearly. Each one (spirit person) has been a different experience because each one of them is different."

This student was learning just how valuable she is to others. She was healing her own old doubts and feelings of unworthiness.

As an intuitive, there is one vital detail that you can do for them . . . calling in transformational specialists to assist them to cross over. Never extend your energy field in order to assist them in crossing over into the Light. Some of my clients have done that and state they were flat in bed for a week. I informed them that this is real, and they journeyed so close to death that they became terribly depleted. Always call in divine and sacred specialty guides to escort a spirit to the best, best place for the spirit's transformation into the Light.

As an intuitive, this will be the most serene, stunningly beautiful event that your intuitive skills allow you to witness. Be ready to observe the greatest moment of healing that you can ever imagine. It will be beautiful beyond anything you can imagine. At first, when you witness this glorious luminescent event you will think you just imagined it. You have not imagined it. Feel and sense the beauty of the moment and how the air literally changed all around you. Feel the difference and know the truth of what just happened.

PART THREE

Confidently Healing Yourself

"Put your ear down close to your soul and listen hard."
—Anne Sexton, *Live or Die*

Chapter 12

How Powerful You Really Are

"We are capable of miraculous results by harnessing the power of energy all around us."

—Maryann Kelly

Are You a Weak or Powerful Link?

Are you a weak or powerful link in the system of the Universe? I hope you are becoming a more powerful link. I hope you are really feeling it more and more. We humans are capable of the most incredible and often miraculous achievements. We are already wired to function at what some would call supernatural abilities. The following list depicts some of our natural human abilities and potentials:

Telepathy – You have the ability to send and receive thought energy between living humans, deceased humans, animals, spirit guides of all types, and nonhuman beings.

Astral Projection – You have the ability to stretch your energy to distant places around the earth and beyond.

Remote Viewing – You have the ability to stretch your energy outward to seek and view objects at a distance.

Laser Beaming – You have the ability to create an intense beam of energy to view within your physical body, (and also others with permission), to receive intuitive medical information.

Manifesting – You have the ability to deliberately direct your own life to actively receive from the Universe.

Uploading and Downloading Intuitive Information – You have the ability to receive and send accurate information from Source.

Perceive Non-physical Beings – You have the ability to see and interact with beings from many non-physical realms.

Healing Yourself and other Humans – You have the ability to create illness in your body and you also have the ability to create healing. You have the ability to alter, heal, and release burdens that lead to your illness and struggles as well as those of other humans.

Healing People in Spirit – You have the ability to communicate with and counsel the deceased to heal their burdens and wounds.

Transitioning People in Spirit – You have the ability to direct specialty guides to escort spirit people into the Light.

Healing Non-humans – You have the ability to perceive, communicate, and direct other types of beings to release the earth plane, release their grip on living or deceased humans.

Transitioning Non-humans – You have the ability to direct specialty guides to escort non-humans into the Light.

Ability to Heal the Past and the Present – You have the ability to heal across time and space. We can heal within the present time frame as well as send healing to the past. Any healing expands into the future.

Traveling to Other Realms – You have the ability to travel to other planets and beyond.

Healing Across Any Distance – You do not need to have your hands on someone, and you accomplish healings from the other side of your city or on the other side of the world.

Did this list just terrify you? Are you terrified to be powerful? You are just as powerful as I am, and other people are just as powerful as you and me. You are in charge of every single moment of your life. You make choices every split second of your life. You and I are all living and learning and then learning some more.

What Does Healing Truly Mean?

I have come up with two significant ways to measure or define healing:

- Releasing of something that is a burden.
- Receiving a lasting positive effect.

When healing has happened your journey will continue to ebb and flow, but the waves will no longer have rough highs like tidal waves do and the lows will not plunge into the depths. The contrast will be less volatile and greatly diminished. The positive and the negative will continue because the earth plane is based on contrast, choices, and decisions. But when you have truly allowed and received significant healing, your boat will not rock so severely. The ebb and flow of life will continue but more like gentle ripples on a lake in the early morning.

Medical Intuition is the ability to receive extremely accurate information regarding your physical body, your emotions, your thoughts, and your life patterns that are creating struggles or illness in your life. The medical intuitive is also the healer for oneself.

You have been learning how to heighten your intuitive skills. Now let's explore healing for you and you alone. It is time for you to recognize the healer within you now, be more in charge of all aspects of your life, create immediate healing experiences for yourself, and learn to master your life and soul. You are now much more in charge of your commands to spirit, but now you are also much more in charge of your own body, thoughts, emotions, and your soul.

It occurred to me that I could create a command to learn in different positive ways and still continue to learn just as much and just as profoundly. This command just flowed into my mind. I was directed by my divine and sacred guides to share it with you:

Teach me to learn more through positive specialty guides of wisdom.
Teach me to learn more through positive physical, mental, and emotional health.
Teach me to learn more through positive life experiences.
Teach me to learn more through positive dream experiences.
Teach me to learn more through positive powerful relationships with the Universe.

This command came to me while I took my morning walk. Just as the words finished going through my mind, a vulture came toward me, flying very low. It tilted its wings just a bit to make sure it flew directly over my head. It came from the east and flew to the west. Now remember that vultures do not represent death. That message in that moment was compelling and intense for me. We may not need to learn from heartache and trauma in life. Let's begin to learn more from positive situations and experiences. The garbage in my life is cleared, cleaned, and carried away. I am learning so much more from the beautiful in life. I want this for you as well . . .

Most people think that painful events of the past have happened and there is absolutely nothing that can be done about it. People are absolutely convinced that emotional and traumatic events will always remain weighty burdens that must be carried throughout this lifetime. That is absolutely not true!

In the following chapters I hope to describe many healing methods in detail so you can understand: 1) energy has no limits, 2) the greatest healing of all happens at an energetic level and not the physical level, and 3) true healing spans out in all directions and crosses time and space.

Stop Now and Notice Yourself with Fascination

Notice what has been popping into your personal thoughts about weighty burdens you are carrying. Whatever pops is always the most genuine. How would you possibly change if you released old, old burdens and traumas? Remember . . . the powerful healer is really you and always has been. What pops into your awareness about that?

My Own Near-Death Experience

I died in New Zealand in 2016. My body was not cured, and yet I had the most precious experience of healing take place within me and throughout me. The near-death experience, in itself, was the most precious healing I could have ever received. I will never be the same. It is so very important to share with you that healing really is releasing burdens and receiving something lighter and of genuine significance.

I was back in my hospital room after the second surgery on my infected hip. I was septic. The infection was throughout my body. I looked up at the ceiling and then the ceiling was gone. I moved forward through a white mist or cloud-like substance. I saw the faces of many, many people, none of whom I knew. We looked deeply but gently into each other's eyes as I passed. I drifted past babies and older people and people of all ages. I stopped for some reason and looked into the eyes of an elderly man. I remained with him for a short period of time as if I was examining him more closely. His eyes suddenly began to glow a menacing, bright red. He was trying to be scary or even evil, but I just laughed and laughed, and then I moved on. I moved past vague formations and still more people and faces.

My drifting slowly came to a stop. I could not go any farther, so I remained standing or sort of floating there. Brilliant colors surrounded me. The lights were so bright it was like I placed my face an inch in front of a multicolored neon sign. My eyes seemed to burn out of my head, but there was no pain at all. The colors continued to hover all around me.

I began laughing with all my heart and could not stop laughing. Laughing so joyously just made me laugh some more. I felt so completely consumed with joy and elation that I had never felt before. I could hear myself laughing. The sounds echoed all around me. My laughter bounced off the wall of colors while some echoed within the colors. My own laughter bounced back to me from all directions like friendly echoes.

As I watched the neon colors, I noticed the brightest light of all was white, and it appeared ahead of me and a little over to my right. The white light blinded me but without pain. The colors formed complicated geometric shapes. The shapes fit tightly together like puzzle pieces. Then the shapes changed and became one shape that duplicated itself. The shapes changed into a multiple of other shapes. I remember one of a tree that duplicated and each duplication fit with itself and repeated all around me. And then the form of a bird duplicated in the same way. I began to laugh more loudly than before. I was truly ecstatic. I was elated, and then I was in my hospital bed again.

The following information comes from the observations and experiences of three medical intuitives. I will call them Chris, Lola, and Mark. According to Google, Chris and Lola live 8,419 miles away from me. The third medical intuitive, Mark, is also a scientist and lives an hour from me. Mark did not know that Chris and Lola were working on me at the same time he was. Chris and Lola live about three hours apart from each other and were not together as they worked with me. All three, however, did medical intuition and supported me energetically while my third surgery was taking place.

Chris tuned into me during the surgery. This was her experience:

"When we started the healing, I saw a Light surgeon come from the Light and enter the body of the real surgeon. When he opened you he pondered for a second on what bits to do. He got a shiver down his spine and then made the decision. It was awesome to watch.

"Next thing was the comment from you about your bum. I turned and you were out of your body. I saw it happening on my left-hand side. I said, 'What are you doing out?' You said, 'I don't know, but I can float.' You started floating on the ceiling and then said, 'Let's go visit a place.' I thought, 'We can't.' We (both medical intuitives) had our (energetic) hands on you doing the healing. Then suddenly a double of ourselves came out. There was a double of Lola, me. I was left to heal, and the second duplicate of us went with you.

"You were floating on top of the surgery room having a laugh. You said, 'I hope my bum isn't sore after this.' You wanted to visit an ancient Pleiadian disc. That's when we found ourselves on a disc meditating. It was a see-through disk with ancient symbols on it. We all sat on it and meditated. We had to tie a white cord on your leg and pull you back into the room and make you heavy so you sunk back in. You were having too much fun and wanted to go to visit other places.

"We (the two medical intuitives) knew you were light and wanted to go places. You were floaty. You wanted to go through a star gate and other places. Thank God for the white cord. We will keep it on until you are better. You were tremendously happy. I started the healing at 10:30 p.m. and it was 2:35 a.m. when I was back in my bed."

Lola also later described the experience she had as she sent healing energy my way.

"You were laughing and had to be pulled back into the room and into your body with a white cord. It was like a comedy . . .

us convincing you we had to go back, and you were sort of on laughing gas and also worried about your bum."

Mark reported this:

"The morning of your surgery, I woke super early and felt strongly that I needed to work on keeping your silver cord attached. It wasn't easy either. I had trouble getting that done. In summary, it was my intention to monitor you throughout your last surgery and broadcast accordingly. The area I found that was most important to address while the surgery was underway pertained to keeping the silver cord attached. The cord can loosen via operations, accidents, drugs, falls, etc. The cord loosening is part of the dying process. It is quite possible that had your silver cord actually loosened you might not have returned to your physical body after the surgery.

It was well after the surgery that your partner told me about the two people in New Zealand who were concurrently working to do the same thing I was attempting to do during the same surgery via different techniques. It was also well after the surgery that you told me that you had the very distinct sense, just prior to surgery, you were not going to make it through that surgery. I had no knowledge of either of these events (the other two healers) as I was attempting the work at that time."

I am told by my guides that I was supposed to have that death experience to teach four truths to humans regarding their innate abilities and supernatural empowerment with life in the non-physical worlds.

1. To help other people remove all fear of releasing their own physical body at the time of death.

2. To assist humans to realize that death is truly an adventure into a more expanded life.

3. To help others awaken and expand their personal comprehension of what reality is really comprised of.

4. To help others learn about the parallel experiences that

my three intuitive companions had. Their experiences demonstrate the ethereal abilities that humans naturally have to venture in, throughout and across time and across the wide, wide spaces.

We are spirits within a spirit world. We are non-physical and physical at same time. You and I, and all humans, are an energetic force, more powerful and more effective in compelling, even magical ways. There is much more going on in the non-physical worlds . . . and we humans on this physical earth are simply part of the whole.

Chapter 13

Twelve Keys to Constantly Do for Yourself

"Nothing is more important than to feel good. And I am going to find ways to do so today."
—Esther Hicks, *Ask and it is Given: Learning to Manifest Your Desires*

1. Save Yourself First

I have tried to save people physically, mentally, emotionally, and spiritually for decades. But I discovered that I had to also save myself along the way. You must save yourself as well. When I tell you to take care of yourself, what comes to your mind? Are you giving to yourself at least equally to the level you give to others? You do not need to give more to yourself, it is vital that you give to yourself equally. What would giving to yourself equally look like in your personal life? Can you do it and will you do it?

2. You are Your Own Healer

I offered medical intuitive readings for many years. I did not realize, until I began to study myself, that my sessions always included a healing. As I studied myself more, the second thing I realized was that I always included the client in every healing that took place. I did this because we are our own healer. The deepest and most permanent healing always included the person participating in their own process.

3. You are One Unit

Most people are so busy with thoughts, they often forget that there is more to them than random, busy thoughts. You are so much more than a thinking machine. Your unit includes your body, thoughts, emotions, and the energy field of your soul. What happens in your thoughts happens in your body at the same time.

4. Do Not Absorb the Energy of Others

Absorbing the negative emotions of others only adds to the negative emotions. It does not assist you or anyone else. Holding the greatest light will not only hold you at a healthier level, it will allow you to be a guide for others.

5. Deliberately Direct Your Toroidal Field

Science has found that energy follows your thoughts. Get in charge of your field. See yourself as a fountain of rainbows, gold, diamond-like sparkles, and then fill yourself with a clear, shimmery, violet flame. Cleanse, brighten up to your maximum, shine from inside outward, and shimmer in the powerful violet flame. Be the best you can be for you.

6. Take the Pop of Intuitive Wisdom

Your thinking mind may seem to be in charge, but just because it is louder and busier, it does not mean it is in charge. Intuitive information pops in as if it comes out of nowhere. The logical thinking mind just keeps chattering on, trying to figure things out.

7. X-Ray Your Body and Field

Healing yourself depends on keeping aware of yourself. Look for weakened areas on a daily basis. It is the same as taking a daily shower. You check out the dusty, dirty places and then scrub your physical body. Now you are also cleaning your energy field and powering up for the day . . . all at the same time!

8. Deliberately Repair Your Energy Field

Scan your field and take charge. Remove negative interference. Deliberately imagine filling rainbows, diamonds, gold, and a violet flame in its place.

Stay quickly and positively in charge. Power Up!

9. Release and then Attract

1) Always remove and release the negative from your energy field.

2) Always and quickly fill the space where the negative used to be, with the highest thoughts and the brightest light of your toroidal field. (See the command under Stop Cutting Cords Now!)

Example commands:

My most holy and sacred Warriors of the Light . . . Completely and permanently remove all negativity from my body, mind, and energy field now. Keep all negativity away from me and keep me away from all negativity.

I am so full of blinding light of Love that only the positive stands with me and everything else is repelled by me now.

10. You are Not Alone

Remember, you are the head of your divine and sacred team of specialists who specialize in you.

11. Trust Yourself and Trust the Specialists

Trust is a mix of thoughts and emotions. Those thoughts and emotions open a smooth, open highway to receive the clearest intuitive wisdom from your specialty guides. They truly are the experts.

12. Take Healing Action Just for You

The deepest healing takes place within the energetic spheres . . . then the physical spheres naturally follow. Equally care for yourself as you take care of others.

Stop Now and Notice Yourself with Fascination

Can you even imagine attending to your own well-being this much or at this degree? Imagine it now and experience the general sensations of the more effective and stronger you.

Chapter 14

Energetic Alerts: What Not to Do

"Every time you don't follow your inner guidance,
you feel a loss of energy, loss of power, a sense of
spiritual deadness."

—Shakti Gawain, *Living in the Light*

Energy Cannot be Killed

So many healers proudly tell me that they got rid of negative dead people or negative entities by killing them. They supposedly kill them by stabbing them with energetic swords, spears, or impaling them with bright light, and so on. Science states in the First Law of Thermodynamics, that one cannot create or destroy energy. One can only transfer it or change it from one form to another. My guides strongly directed me to never attempt to kill a negative being of any kind. So . . . I don't. I call in transitional specialists to take the being to the highest place for its transformation into Light and Love. (Much more on this later in this book.)

Never Chase Spirit People or Non-Humans Away

Dead people and other types of entities are real. They are real beings even if they are not physical at the moment. If you try to kill them, or in this case, chase them away, they have to go somewhere else. New mentoring clients often tell me that they find negative beings interfering with their clients. Then they tell me how they successfully chased them away. As they tell me their stories, I intuitively see what happens. I see the deceased people or other types of beings literally leap into the client themselves or I see the beings run out of the house and into the neighbor's house. They have to go somewhere because they are real and need to have a location. (Precise steps to assist beings to transform is later in this book.)

Stop Cutting Energy Cords Now!

I teach my workshops all over the world. My goal all around the globe is to teach energy healers and practitioners on all levels to stop cutting cords. When I declare that to a crowd, someone usually calls out, "We have got to cut them, or they will stay connected and negatively affect people!" Cords are real, but cutting cords is not the solution!

Picture this . . . I am holding one end of a garden hose and you hold the other end. A well-meaning healer comes by and cuts the garden hose somewhere in between us. I am still holding one piece of it and you are holding the other piece. We are both still affected by the hose because we are both still holding it as we go on with our individual life. In other words, nothing was healed. Here is an example of an energy healer struggling to understand energetic cords and what to do about them.

Client: We talk a lot about what to do when working with clients. What do I do if I am feeling off? What do we do if it is us and we are in panic mode?

TZ: You know that you are saying this right now and it is not just because you do not feel well right now. You are also bringing it up because I just began writing my fifth book which is about doing this level of work for ourselves! Look how intuitive you are. How long have you not been feeling well?

Client: It's funny. I began feeling anxiety several months ago and

I am not an anxious person, but I have been doing a lot of energy work lately. Well, it's just a feeling, so I decided it was just because I am feeling more than before.

TZ: No. That should not cause anxiety because you are doing more energy work.

Client: Well, yesterday I thought, 'Am I having an anxiety attack?' My blood pressure was pounding. My body was freaking out. I felt like my heartbeat was coming out of my skin. Pulse rate was really fast. My blood pressure is normally very, very low and it has been high. I do not have high blood pressure. In fact, it is typically low. I have also been working on myself for about a year. Now, if I work on myself to see what is going on with me personally, how do I find or see or know what is going on with me?

TZ: Here is what I would say, first of all. Have you been energetically removing yourself from clients you have been working with?

Client: No.

TZ: When we work with others at this level for another person we are creating an unusual connection with other people. There are cords and threads and connections with our family and friends that are very positive. But when we work with others on an energetic level we are creating an intense cord to another person. If we do not remove that cord, that intensity, we are still affected by every single person we have ever worked with. We are also talking about our coworkers and other people we have worked with.

Client: Oh my gosh, that makes so much sense!

TZ: It makes sense because you are saying that you do not feel like yourself. (When you or someone you know uses those words, it is an intuitive signal or piece of information about yourself and a key to knowing that some type of negative interference might be happening).

Client: This makes so much sense because the client I am working with right now has been saying, "I do not know where all this anxiety is coming from."

TZ: Your client's anxiety is coming to you from her. What I want you to ask for is a sacred, divine specialty guide who excels in creating cleansing filters to come forward for you now. Always use the word "now" because spirit is very "airy fairy" about time. Using the word now tends to send a strong signal to them. Always say now.

Also using the words "divine" and "sacred" sends out a high frequency and vibration, so you do not get just anybody. You want the best. We could create our own filters, but I am telling you it will not be better than what a specialty guide can create for us. When I began doing this and bringing me back to myself through the cleaning filter there would be black slime or chunks of stuff hanging on the filter (that was negative energy from the people I was helping). I wanted to bring the purest and cleanest back to me. If we do not do this we can still bring ourselves back to us, but there will be residual energy from the client's crap in their life or body that we might bring back to us. I have worked with thousands of people, and if I did not do this I would be dead by now or crazy in a nursing home.

The command that I give my cleansing filter specialty guide is this: *I bring me and only me back to myself clean and clear through the filter provided for me, and I bring me back to myself through the filter from every single person I have ever worked with.*

When I added the part, "and from every single person I have ever worked with," body parts and faces came out of me for three weeks or more. I know I was going back in time releasing all the negative connections with others in my life.

You need this command right now and you need to do it repeatedly.

Client: Yes, I want to write it down. (She wrote it down exactly as I stated it). I have not been removing myself. I didn't know this.

TZ: Hardly anyone does, and I am teaching all over the world trying to tell people about this healing technique.

Even if you are not a healing practitioner, you still may have negative cording that either you sent to another person or someone sent to you. Anger or negative thoughts about another person deliberately or unconsciously create negative cords.. In either case, the cord should never be cut. It needs to be removed and not cut. That is a massive difference.

Steps to Remove Negative Cords:

1. Call out for a divine and sacred guide who specializes in removing negative cords. Pause and allow yourself to notice or sense the guide who arrives.

2. Notice the direction the cord seems to be flowing. In other words, did you create it and send it to the other person, or did someone connect in with you?

3. Clearly command the following to the specialist if someone else corded into you:
   Completely and permanently remove every root, every particle of the negative cord out of my body, my mind, my spirit, and my soul now! Completely transform it into divine, unconditional love and send it back to the person who sent it now!

4. Call out for your divine and sacred healing specialist and command:
   Completely and permanently fill every single space and place where that negativity used to be with vitality, cellular health, unconditional love.

5. You must actively participate with your specialists to allow the healing to happen and also to actively receive the goodness to come into you.

Take note: Not all cords are negative. Each of us has the "silver cord" at the base of our spine. The silver cord is the positive connection between the body and our soul or higher self. You may recognize the reference from earlier in my in my friend's accounts during my near-death experience.

Here is a quote from a well-known radionics lecturer and intuitive consultant, Caroline Connor:

> "The silver cord that is attached to the end of your tailbone keeps you in your body. At night you astro-travel in your dreams. The cord brings you back to your human body or shell. When it becomes loose and dangles up and down, the need to leave the body is very strong and produces thoughts of suicide. When the cord is reattached, the desire to die leaves. You are working with the seat of the WILL TO LIVE. This cord can become loose through surgeries, accidents, drugs, and falls. (The cord becoming loose is a natural process of dying.) When the cord is loose, HOPELESSNESS sets in, so you must replace this emotion with HOPEFULNESS."

Other positive cords naturally occur between our family members and friends who we care about. It is actually more difficult to perceive positive cords because they are so light in nature while negative cords will look dark, sometimes thick. The darker and thicker it appears will tell you that it has been there longer.

Do Not Pray Against Something or Someone

A prayer is a command, but it is a gentle command for Source, or the Universe, or God to do something about something or someone. Prayers, especially prayers that you are deeply feeling become a thing of substance going out into the Universe. If you pray or command against someone or something, then you are also adding to the negative situation that is happening.

Never deliberately send negative thought energy to another person. Always be careful with your words even if you distinguish it as a prayer. Word the prayer in all positive words and direct it to the positive that you want. Here is an excerpt of two people praying or commanding, in such a sincere way. They did not realize they were commanding to receive the negative words they were sending outward:

Client: Freedom comes into my mind. I do not want negative words to impact me so much. I am very aware that these are things that I do not need to worry about any more . . . I do mindset journaling every morning when I do meditation and breath work. I want to be free from their impact. I even journal things every day like, "I do not feed fear . . . I do not feed fear . . . I do not feed fear." I do that because I have allowed things to build up.

TZ: You are commanding to the Universe: Feed my fear! That is what the Universe is really picking up from your command. You never want to use the words that describe exactly what you are trying to not do, trying to avoid.

Client: Oh, thank goodness, this is so good.

TZ: You said you are stating this every day, and you are smashing yourself down every day! My guides have been telling me for the last couple of minutes that you self-punish. You are very good at self-punishment. Then you told me that you are commanding every day to feed the fear! Tell me exactly the command you are saying every day.

Client: I say, I *don't* feed fear.

TZ: The Universe does not pick up the "don't." The Universe is neutral, so it says, "Okay, she still wants to feed fears."

Client: No wonder I am! This is monumental!

TZ: Yes! This is monumental. Do not use the very words that you are trying to get rid of in your life. Let's start with this . . . What is the opposite of feeding fear?

Client: Feeding love.

TZ: Yes, something like that. But do you also realize you are commanding the word "feed" which makes the command land in your digestive system. (Earlier in this session, the client told me she was struggling with her digestive system.)

Client: Oh my goodness, I didn't even think of that! This is amazing! And I say it every day. My partner and I are so committed to our spiritual evolution together as a team. We actually both do this. We say every day that we do not feed fear. We say this to each other and we say it to the Universe. And my partner, over this last year has randomly begun to feel nauseous, and his digestion is bothering him. We even have a page that we have our intentions written that we do together.

TZ: I want you two to go through that list or even throw it away. You are commanding with an unbelievable powerful energy, the opposite of what you want.

Essential Points

- Do not chase spirit people away. Treat them as someone in need of something.

- Do not try to kill spirit people because energy cannot be killed, only transformed.

- Never cut cords attached to you or someone else. They must be removed and released for healing to happen.

- Never use the words that describe what you are trying to release or get rid of.

- Never pray against something. Always pray with positive words and positive emotions to make the greatest difference.

Chapter 15

Healing Your History is the Secret Key

"A healer's power stems not from any special ability, but from maintaining the courage and awareness to embody and express the universal healing power that every human being naturally possesses."

—Eric Micha'el Leventhal, *A Light from the Shadows*

This is the most important chapter in this book. The following is indeed the key to permanent healing.

Pills, surgery, all types of health counseling, taking a vacation, supplements, reading more books, or going to more doctors is not going to heal anything at the level I am advocating in this book. For a profound, authentic, and lasting healing to take place you must heal your past first. Your past could be yesterday, three days ago, at the age of five, or it could be over twenty-six lifetimes ago. The length of time is insignificant. But what is overpoweringly significant is where the healing needs to be directed. Healing must be directed to the point where it all began.

No More Bandages

Have you ever heard the old saying in counseling that healing is like peeling the layers from the onion . . . one layer at a time, ever so slowly? Those "peeling away" techniques are not only slow, but is anything ever completely healed and released in the process? Physically-based healing techniques are supportive and sometimes absolutely necessary like surgery for an injury or going to the emergency room at a hospital for an actual emergency, removing a cancerous tumor, getting lab tests to have a measurement of the situations going on in the body.

We are blessed to have Western medicine. Integrative medicine is the combination of Western medicine and alternative health techniques all working together and are all needed in the physical world. But there is more that lies hidden beneath these physical conditions, illnesses, and struggles. What lies there is the "cause." There is always something that causes repetition of illness, negative patterns, emotional stress, and strife. For the depth of healing to take place, you must direct the healing to the point where it all started: in other words, the exact cause.

This transcription offers an example of a physical-level struggle lasting forty-three years, but it stopped when the cause was healed.

"No allergy shots needed after forty-three years! The red, scaly eczema rash that covered my body was the immediate visual sign that I was an infant plagued with allergies. If that weren't enough of an indication, my piercing screams echoing off the walls in our tiny row home caused a visceral reaction among the five others in my home as well as in the neighbors' homes, sharing common walls, adjacent on either side of our home.

"The standard physician prescribed infant formula to use in replacement of mother's milk, and it exacerbated the eczema which covered me head to toe as an infant. My immune system produced additional allergic manifestations by severe allergies to grasses, trees, and pollen. Elementary school brought new challenges associated with playmates who had pets, as I found that I was allergic to common pets. Then they cautioned me regarding foods as well to avoid an allergic reaction. Childhood, for me, had hallmarks of itchy eyes, a running nose, and my head felt so heavy from constant sinus congestion.

"When I was fifteen years old, I was tested for over a hundred allergens across categories of trees, grasses, pollens, animals, dust mites, mold, and foods. I was so overall highly allergic that what were to be individual and discretely separate tiny red spots indicating the degree of a reaction produced a large, extremely itchy welt covering my back. Within minutes, I had difficulty breathing and my eyes swelled closed as the allergic reaction became systemic throughout my body.

"The goal was to have a customized serum of three injections every one to three weeks all year round, and I was desensitized to the many elements that I was allergic to. At thirty years old, I wanted to see if I could possibly do without them. Being off these shots proved disastrous, and so I gratefully relented and went back to my allergy injection regimen. When I was thirty-one years old, I was transferred to work in the United Kingdom from the United States. Because of my specialized need for my highly customized allergy shots, I had to pursue private health care alternatives in the United Kingdom via the American Embassy.

"Part of my (healing) journey involved connecting with loved ones who have crossed over and holistic health with medical intuition. I was fascinated to learn about techniques that could address even chronic conditions. I found that the techniques I had learned from Tina Zion were most effective with my clients. I wanted to apply these techniques to my allergies, not only to get symptomatic relief but also to effectively address the associated root cause.

"Once I could identify and address the energetic root cause, the goal was to no longer need these shots, and I would have my own testimonial regarding 'walking the walk.' I began by identifying the point of origin associated with my allergies and found that the point of origin was associated with a past life. During the associated past life regression, I faced that past life point of origin which had triggered my autoimmune reaction as manifested by allergies. I brought the associated resolution forward to the current time as consistent with Tina's modality.

"Concurrent with the above step, I also wrote and followed an individualized dowsing script based upon Raymon Grace's methodology as Tina had taught. Along with the above steps, Tina had introduced me to Epigenetics, so I read books by Dr. Bruce Lipton and Dr. Joe Dispenza. I envisioned my future free of needing allergy shots. The body does, indeed, believe what it is told. I had been told I was a victim to genetics, doomed to allergies. I told my body, and I believed that a different future was attainable. Within a few weeks, I was forgetting that I hadn't had an allergy shot in weeks. This was shocking.

"In February 2020, I was due for the next comprehensive test of approximately one hundred allergens across the same categories. To my delight, there was such a minimal to negligible reaction to the same many allergens during this test that my physician, specializing in immunotherapy and allergies, who had known me for many years, was quite surprised. The entire test was repeated. I no longer needed any allergy shots! I had gone from forty-three years needing allergy shots with three injections at each visit to no shots. Now I am my own testimonial that this process of self-healing works! We are all capable of miraculous results by harnessing the power of energy all around us. I am so grateful to Tina for her guidance and mentorship."

Healing at the physical level is cumbersome and inhibited by the dense nature of the physical realm. An everlasting healing has more opportunity to take place on an energetic level because energy has no boundaries. To put the most incredible healing into action, we must go to the exact point where the illness originated. If we do not discover that exact instant, our efforts to heal will tend to be more superficial. In other words, each physical, mental, or emotional illness has a precise origin.

That point of origin is the foundation and direct cause of the illness or issue. If we do not get to the precise cause of the disease or struggle, our healing efforts will be somewhat superficial and temporary. To have an original cause implies that something happened in the past. Again remember, the past could be back centuries ago or just yesterday. So the cause could be anything, happen anywhere and at any time. It is often a moment that you have no awareness about. There is one very important and constant factor involved, however. The moment of cause is always riddled with intense emotions. The intensity of raw emotions creates an immense force of energy. That mighty force of emotional energy travels across time and space and often does not seem to weaken as time goes on.

How to Find the Exact Cause of Your Illness and Struggles

A violin instructor just retired from teaching in the school system but soon decided to teach children in their homes as a part-time career. This was going along quite well for a short time until she plunged off a client's front porch and shattered her arm. She just completed teaching the three children in that home for the first time. This is a good example of an accident when there is really no such thing as an accident.

Rather than attempting to figure out the cause of this event with my rational, logical thinking mind, I took a very different approach. I asked in a commanding way to be given the exact point of origin that caused (her name) fractured arm. I clairvoyantly perceived the answer in my mind's eye. As a child this woman lived in agony with an alcoholic father and a terrified, abused mother. Her primary memory was loud fighting and beatings. As a child and as an adult, she had thought everyone lived this way. But then she found herself at the age of sixty teaching the violin in a home of a gentle, loving family. Spirit said that this literally knocked her off her feet. It was as if the earth shook beneath her, knocked her off balance, and rocked her world. Now she knew the true cause of falling off their steps and shattering her arm. This is information that an X-ray could never reveal. This is the beginning of healing at the point of origin causing the "accident."

Discovering the inception point of any illness or injury is so simple that you will insist that there must be more to it than this. You turn it over to your guides. Call out to your specialists in a commanding manner, asking for the exact point that a certain malady began. Be specific with your request. Do not just call out for help. Our words create energy, so we must be careful how we phrase what we want and for whom we want it. Here are some examples of statements that will prompt the specialty guides to provide the most accurate information for you:

The following command is direct and effective. You must always send this command to your most sacred and divine guides. And for your health and well-being, call out to your divine and sacred medical intuitive guides and invite them in. You must really mean it when you command it and then be ready for the answer and be ready that you might be in for a surprise:

Tell me or show me now the exact point of origin that caused (name the illness/struggle) for me, (your full name).

Pause and take the pop.

You will receive the information in thoughts, images, or little movies showing in your mind's eye. Then you must be ready for surprises. These insights will take you to one of eight categories of causes that are described in the last section of this book.

Heal Your Past, Present, and Future Now

This is an account of one woman's description of events that led to her own stunning healing. Notice that she describes multiple causes of her physical illness. Also notice they are all in her past.

"Early in the year, I went to the gynecologist for an annual checkup. During the examination she pointed out that I had two small cysts around one to 1.5 centimeters growing on the left ovary. When I asked the doctor why they were there, she replied, 'Sometimes it happens.' This explanation wasn't satisfactory, so I started to reattach and explore the metaphysical meaning behind the cyst. Anything that is happening in our bodies is a physical manifestation of what is going on mentally, emotionally, or spiritually. After reading about how unprocessed trauma can be stored in our bodies, I went to work on healing. I did a six-hour body immersion session followed by three womb healings and a chakra alignment.

"When I returned to the doctor for another examination on Friday afternoon, I asked her if she could perform another ultrasound to check on the cyst. She was short on time and not overly happy with the request but went ahead with it anyway. You could imagine the shock when she told me the two small cysts had now grown into one big cyst almost seven centimeters in size. She requested that I make an appointment immediately to be operated on and have the cysts removed. I called the clinic and was booked in on Monday for another scan, and then they wanted to operate on the following Tuesday.

"I arrived at the clinic, and they confirmed that, yes, there was a cyst almost seven centimeters, and it would be in my best interest to go ahead with the operation on the following Tuesday. I asked if they would check again to see if the cyst had changed in size prior to the operation in which they replied, no they would not. With a week before the operation, I organized another appointment on the Monday night before the operation. That's when I called Tina.

"Tina politely asked if she could take a look (I looked into her abdomen). We landed at (the memory) of the passing of my granny. Up until this point, I didn't realize that there were any stored emotions in relation to this. Of all my grandparents, and actually all the people in the world, Granny was my favourite person. When she was sick, my family sent me away to stay at a friend's place. When I returned, they told me she had passed away. I was devastated, and I felt betrayed; however, I suppressed all this so I could look 'strong for my family.'

"The second part had to do with the fact that when I was a young girl, my grandfather asked my grandmother to leave the room, and then he went on to abuse me. I had done so much healing regarding the abuse, but I had never realized again that, deeply imbedded in me, was the feeling of betrayal. In both cases, Tina led me through a soul retrieval to heal the past.

"Part (of my health issues) had to do with my own mother who was an alcoholic. One night she had too much to drink and fell back on a huge painting we had and smashed her head on the glass. The glass shattered everywhere, and my mother then fell down to the ground and slumped over. Again, Tina led me through a Soul retrieval to heal the past.

"On Monday, I arrived at the doctor, and she asked me to explain why I was there. I told her I had the operation scheduled tomorrow, and they wouldn't do an ultrasound before the surgery. I wanted to check and see if there were any changes. Completely irritated at my request, the doctor went ahead with the ultrasound, only to confirm that there was absolutely no cyst."

I studied the methods and steps that my guides directed me to teach people how powerful and capable they are, and how they are meant to heal themselves. The next section describes eight categories of cause, and the healing methods that consistently have powerful results for people. Every time an intense, permanent healing has taken place, I am aware that four factors are in action:

1. The intent to become healed is focused, deliberate, and commanding.

2. The person feels powerful and invincible while the information and the energy of Source flows through them.

3. The person has an absolute, unshakable knowing that they are now in charge of their own energy field and their own thoughts.

4. Each person allows the healing to happen and allows a complete release of the old trauma or suffering.

All the qualities of healing, at the energetic level, steadily ripple throughout time and space. Healing ripples and vibrates within your body, mind, and soul and outward throughout relationships, your environment, and into every aspect of your life.

Essential Points

- Heal your history first.
- Much that we consider healing is merely a bandage.
- Direct all your healing to the cause beneath the illness or struggle.
- Causes of your illness or struggles are in your past.
- Healing at the energetic level steadily ripples throughout time and space and your life.

PART FOUR

Eight Primary Causes & Your Action Steps to Heal

"Stay humble . . . Stay listening to others and to
your own heart . . . Stay loving . . . Because everyone
around you is broken in some way . . . but that just
allows God's Light to shine through all the cracks!"

—My Aunt Donna, 90 Years of Wisdom

Up to now, this book has focused on excelling as an intuitive and
a medical intuitive. Using precise steps, you have been observing,
studying, and learning about the intuitive you along the way. I
have defined specific steps and processes to rocket your intuitive
skills to be a powerful and extraordinarily competent intuitive.
Your intuitive awareness includes the physical and the non-
physical realms. You have learned that you are more than a body
with a thinking head on top of it. You have discovered how to
scan your body and energy field for intrusive energy and how to
power up your field from the inside outward rather than create a
barrier around you. We discussed that healing your history is the
fundamental and crucial element for a complete and permanent
healing.

The last portion of this book focuses on finding the exact cause of your illness, repetitive issues, and struggles. I have witnessed over and over again that the cause generally groups into eight different categories. Finding the direct cause of your struggles is so simple that you may not believe it will even work, or that it is even real. It works and it is real. It works because you have purposefully enriched and advanced your intuitive abilities and deepened your trust of the divine and sacred specialty guides along the way. Now you can take the next action that will take you to the exact cause of your struggles or illness you have been grappling with throughout some portion of your life.

The following command is direct and effective. Do not send this command out to the general Universe. You must always send this command to your most sacred and divine medical intuitive guides. You must really mean it when you command it and then be ready for the answer when it pops! You must trust the pop and do not push it aside as your imagination or fantasy. It might, however, be a surprise or something you have always known.

The steps are:

1. Invite your divine and sacred medical intuitive guides to come and work with you.

2. State this command to the guide: *Tell me or show me now the exact point of origin that is causing me, (your full name) to have (name the illness/struggle/issue).*

3. Split second of a pause . . .

4. Receive the answer in thoughts, pictures, and little movies in your mind's eye.

5. Your guide's answer will tell you in words, or show you in pictures or movies, the exact moment that a particular struggle/illness began. The information you just received generally fall into one of the eight categories.

The categories of cause are:

1. Your Thoughts and Emotions.

2. Your Physical Body Needs

3. Your Current Life Traumas and Losses

4. Your Relationships with Family and Friends

5. Your Environment

6. Your Past Life Traumas and Losses

7. Your Ancestors

8. The Non-physical Spirit Realms

Some of the information in Part Four will be a repeat from earlier portions of this book. The difference is now, we are looking at these things as the cause of your illness or issues. Each of the following eight chapters describes one cause and specific methods to heal and permanently release the cause.

Remember . . . permanent healing has happened when you feel a complete release of emotions about the cause. The cause turns into neutral information that no longer carries any impact inside of you. Energetic healings create ripples of positive change in all directions within your body and mind. Healing at the energetic level sends delicate, buoyant ripples across time and space and into your eternal soul.

Chapter 16

Cause #1: Your Thoughts and Emotions

"Your pain is the breaking of the shell that encloses
your understanding."
—Khalil Gibran, *The Prophet*

Thoughts and Emotions are Beneath All Issues

The most dramatic cause of our diseases, illnesses, and issues is
our thoughts and subsequent emotions. You are your thoughts.
Your thoughts and emotions are either harming you or healing
you. I discussed this in my book, *Become a Medical Intuitive*, but it
is so important that I will briefly discuss it again here. Remember,
science has discovered that energy follows human thoughts. Each
word within our thoughts and our requests has its own vibration
and will attract things from the Universe that are of a similar
vibration. You are the only one who is really in charge of you. You
are the only one who can decide to learn, advance, expand, hide,
shrink, follow old rules that do not feel right, make new friends,
and the list goes on and on.

No matter what happens in your life, you do not need to think
of it as a mistake if you learn something about yourself from the
situation. You cannot "make up" for your wrongs in your past or
try to make up for who you are. Trying to make up for something
only keeps you in the vibration of being wrong, bad, or negative.
Do not focus on learning about the other people involved either.
True profound awareness is learning about yourself in each

stressful situation. You can then observe everything around you and expand your awareness about how life works and evolves.

Check in with yourself frequently. Emotions crop up in surprising ways and at surprising times. Even some mentoring clients grow concerned as they live a more intuitive life. One very conscientious client felt guilty and blurted out, "I am sitting with people in a restaurant and I suddenly know things about them. I am trying so hard not to be invasive and to honor people's privacy. These people have not given me permission to get intuitive information, but I am getting it anyway. I think it is leading me to being judgmental when I know these things!"

Like so many highly intuitive people, this man was distressed. He felt a great deal of relief when I pointed out that we intuitives will simply know things because we are intuitive. That is different from being invasive into other people's bodies and lives. Had he not attended to this guilt in the moment he might have shut down his intuitive skills that had recently opened.

As you go throughout the days of your life, do it with the clearest awareness and intent. We are designed to be an important component of the Universe. Our bodies, our world, and our Universe become more positive or more negative based on our thought energy.

Your Painful Memories and Your Secrets

When you command to be told or shown the cause of your issues, you will often discover or remember painful memories or secrets. Please be okay to discover and to know about these issues in your life. Negative emotions, painful memories, and secrets are thick and sticky and can make us terribly ill, physically and mentally. Remember that guilt and shame have the lowest vibrations and, as a result, they cause some type of physical or mental challenge or illness. They can actually destroy us at many levels of life. This client shares her experience with healing methods for her physical pain.

"I started having severe jaw pain several years ago due to clenching at night. Although I wore a mouth guard, the pain progressed. I was eventually diagnosed with TMJ. In August 2017 I woke up one morning with terrible jaw pain and unable to open my mouth. I was then diagnosed with disc displacement in my jaw. I was not able to open my mouth more than about one inch, and chewing was painful. I resorted to living on soft foods and smoothies. I went to a Physical Therapist for months and even saw a TMJ specialist with very little relief. I was in pain daily, and my jaw was constantly popping. I was told by two doctors and my physical therapist it may not ever fully heal.

"Fast forward to when I started working together with Tina in 2019. I started using her practices to heal my jaw. I asked my guides to show me the exact point of origin of my jaw pain and found the pain had an emotional cause that needed healing. I went back to be with my younger self and gave back all the negative emotions and took back my power and did a soul retrieval. It was a very emotional journey that provided deep healing and a sense of peace. I continued to do a daily practice of asking my healing specialists to fully heal my jaw and truly believed I would heal.

"After doing the soul retrieval, I began to first notice reduced pain and much less clenching at night. Then I began to notice I could open my mouth wider and wider and chew without pain. As of today, I have *full* range of motion and no pain! I can eat what I want and even bite a giant sandwich! Just more and more evidence of the magic of this work!"

Notice that this client did soul retrieval work, but she also continued to work with her guides and direct them toward what she wanted to accomplish. (More on the soul retrieval steps in Current Life Traumas section.)

Begin now to sense your thoughts and emotions as energy. Are your thoughts and emotions often jagged, knifelike, needles, bullets, sticky, heavy, or have they been bright like a star or the sun? Have they been a cool breeze, strong waves lapping onto a beach, or puffs of bright white clouds or ripples light and airy? Study and translate your thoughts/emotions into different electrical frequencies radiating out from you into the world around you.

Whose Ideas Do You Have—Theirs or Yours?

Whose ideas and beliefs repeat over and over in your mind? Are they truly your original beliefs, or did you swallow someone else's ideas and make them your own? Even as I ask you just now, take the pop of memories. Do you believe that you do not deserve anything in life, or do you believe that you should only go so far and can't achieve the next step because you do not deserve any more? Where and when did your limitations begin? Take the pop right now and notice it as intuitive information.

For the most part, children are not aware of limitations, not aware of feelings of not deserving, do not feel worry or fear, do not naturally feel hate. These are just a few examples of struggles that we hear along the way. We hear it from bullies, parents, grandparents, or authoritative role models. At what point did you swallow their beliefs and make them your own? Take the *pop!*

Just because you might have swallowed someone's low energy ideas does not mean you need to keep them any longer. Sort that out for you and about you. Will you allow yourself to have unlimited ideas of your own? It is up to you.

Forgiveness: New Thoughts About It

Remember that everything is energy and has its own energetic frequency, even forgiveness. First of all, do not tell yourself that you must forgive someone. Do not listen to anyone who tells you that you must forgive. Do not try to forgive others and do not try to forgive yourself either. Forgiveness is not a healing technique. Counselors and friends will tell you that because they do not know what else to say. They are not aware that pushing you to forgive creates more critical judgment towards yourself. It will just make you angry and more resentful, and you end up thinking you are a failure. Again, forgiveness is not a healing technique. You cannot get to forgiveness by someone telling you to forgive or for you to demand it of yourself. It does not create the healing. Healing has to come first. Forgiveness is the natural, effortless result after the healing. It comes after the release of all emotions regarding the situation.

Summary of Action Steps to Heal and Release

1. Learn about you by examining yourself first and not everyone else. Notice everything about your thoughts, emotions, and actions. Focus everything on: What you are learning, could be learning, should be learning from each situation. Learn constantly about yourself and do not focus on learning about others.

2. Throughout the day notice your thoughts and emotions in terms of energy. Is your energy soft, sharp, jagged, inflamed, agitated, conditional or unconditional, cold, loving? Notice the energy without judgment.

3. Do not make forgiveness your goal. Learning and healing is your goal.

4. Whose limitations are inside your mind? Are they really yours? Where did you get them from? Command your guides to remove them from your energy field now.

5. Do not be afraid or judgmental to learn more about yourself. Do not stop now.

Chapter 17

Cause #2: Your Physical Body Needs

"The curious paradox is that when I accept myself
just as I am, then I can change."
—Carl R. Rogers, *On Becoming a Person*

Talk to Your Body, Then Listen!

Yes, your physical body has its own needs. Are you giving your body what it needs? Do you know what it wants or needs? Communicate with your body. Communicate with the disease or illness or painful area. Talk to it exactly like it was another person that you are getting to know and understand in a special way.

Notice other people's language when they struggle with their physical body. They frequently disown that section of their body. For example, instead of saying, "my shoulder," they will say "the shoulder." If you have an illness or struggle, your body is asking for recognition. It does not heal by disowning it. It heals by developing a meaningful relationship with it.

This man in my office was in great physical pain. I asked him to pretend and imagine walking all around the pain. I explained, "It will feel like you are simply making it all up and it will seem like a movie, but go ahead anyway and let's see what happens." I directed him to let his imagination just unfold like a tiny movie in his mind's eye. "Slowly go behind the pain . . . Slowly look above the painful area . . . Now go underneath it . . . Now look all around the pain. Check it out with interest and be fascinated and go with whatever you notice. Describe it to me." I then suggested that he slowly ask the pain these questions and take whatever leaps into his mind without judgment:

- What color are you?
- How big are you?
- What are you made of?
- What emotions are inside of you?
- How long have you been there?
- At what moment did you arrive?

There were heavy emotions deep inside of his upper abdomen (solar plexus). This client asked these questions one at a time. He did not move on to the next question until he noticed whatever picture or words popped into his thoughts and his mind's eye. The pain quickly answered all his questions.

Begin by asking your entire body as a whole some questions and accept whatever leaps, jumps, or pops into your thoughts or mind's eye:

- Where are your struggles located?
- What are you trying to tell me?
- When did this struggle begin?
- What are you trying to learn?
- What are you trying to accomplish?
- What are you refusing to learn?
- Where is that refusal located?
- How did it change us?
- Did we make a mistake?
- Can we learn from mistakes?
- What do we need to learn first?

Now talk directly to the disease, pain, organ, section, or

ailment. Develop a true communication with it and the area it is located within you. Ask these questions, but give it a moment to answer you:

- Why are you in that location of my body?
- Exactly when did you start there?
- What emotions are inside of you?
- What memories are inside of you?
- What do you want me to know about you?
- What secrets have you been keeping from me?
- Tell me what you need to permanently heal and release.

Another client did this process with me. She was discussing the terrible feeling in her chest. She described that she was torn. She said, "It is a struggle inside of me between love versus fear." I asked her to look into her chest and let her body show her an image. She immediately said she sees a net around her heart. I asked her to talk to her heart and ask it specific questions. Examples of good questions might be:

- "Heart . . . When did the net appear all around you?"
- "Heart . . . Why is the net there?"
- "Heart . . . What does the net do for you?"
- "Heart . . . What would happen if together we removed the net?"

Water and Food is Medicine

The earth is approximately 75 percent water. According to H.H. Mitchell in the *Journal of Biological Chemistry*, the human body is about 60 percent water as well. About 73 percent of the organs of the heart and brain is water. Humans are nearly all water. It is a primary factor in body functions such as: regulating body temperature, transporting and metabolizing food into the blood system, releasing waste material in urination, acting as a shock absorber in the brain and spinal cord, forming saliva and the lubrication inside of our joints. We cannot function without it.

Imagine that we deliberately power up our water before we drink it. Then what would happen?

Science has found that water responds to emotions as it also holds the vibrations of emotions. Place hands on a container of water or your food. Imagine creating the energy of love and health, and at the same time create very specific positive thoughts and feelings that apply to you. Maintain those exact same thoughts and positive emotions as you deliberately push all that great and positive energy into the food or water. You will literally eat and drink those vibrations, and those vibrations will absorb throughout the cells of your body. How about drinking and eating powerful vibrations of love for yourself?

Ask and listen to your body regarding food. Ask it questions like:

- What is the best food for you?
- What food do you need the most right now?
- Why do you want that food right now?
- What does that food do for me really?
- Why do I feel terrible when I eat_____?

Also, command to your divine and sacred guides: *Show me or tell me now the exact point of origin causing my struggles about food.* Pause . . . and receive the *pop* of information.

Evaluate Prescriptions and Supplements

A client once asked me if I could tell with my medical intuitive abilities if his medicines and supplements were good for him. I said, "I don't know. Give me a second and let me ask my guides." What I was really saying to my guides is, what the heck can I do about this? Here is what my divine and sacred medical intuitive guides said to me. They said, "Tell him to go get the bottles of his medicines and supplements." So, I told him that, and as he ran off to get them, I said to the guides, "Now what?" They very clearly said to have him hold one bottle at a time and say the name of it out loud to you. You simply watch his energy field and inform him how his energy field responds.

It was amazing to see that some of the supplements and meds dulled his field; some made his energy look like it was caving in on itself while others expanded and brightened his field. As a medical intuitive you never direct anyone to stop any medications or supplements. What we intuitives can do is describe how the body and energy field responds. Intuitives, who do not have a medical license, are not stepping out of bounds when they just describe the energy changes. That is not illegal.

This book is not about doing medical intuition for others, however. This book is about doing healing steps for yourself. Here is a segment from a session where we talked about doing these steps for ourselves.

Client: I have vitamins, and I have a whole thing of vitamins. Sometimes I do not know what is good for me. I was taking one and I think it was making me feel sick. So how do I check in with those things? Do I just ask my guides if this is good for me?

TZ: No. First of all, it is of utmost importance to always use more specific words, more precise words (when communicating with your guides). I want you to hold each supplement or prescription, one at a time, and state the name out loud to your guide with the question such as: *Is (name the supplement/ prescription) excellent for my physical health?* Do you see how much more specific a question that is? Then you must notice what your energy field does and what your guides tell you. Then put it down, write down what you received about it. Then go on to the next one.

Client: Oh, that is good. I am going to practice that technique. This has given me a lift because I have been so frustrated with it (assessing prescriptions and supplements).

Steps to Assess Your Medications and Supplements:

1. Have paper and a pen to log all the details that you receive.

2. Sit in front of a large mirror to notice your own energy field.

3. Use specific, precise words as you question your guides.

4. Call out to your divine and sacred medical intuitive specialist who excels with medications. (This command will assure that you get the guide who is the best with medicines out of your team of guides.)

5. Hold each supplement or prescription, one at a time.

6. Command the following: Tell me or show me now . . . Is (name the supplement / prescription) excellent for my physical health? (Receive the answer.) Does it work positively for me? (Receive the answer.)

7. Notice: What words pop into your mind instantly from your specialist.

   a. Feel your energy field as you command that question.

   b. Watch your field in the mirror.

8. Write down whatever you received and noticed about each medicine and supplement.

Create Your Own Scalar Waves

We discussed earlier how to talk and listen to your body and how to talk and listen to the disease or illness that is happening within you. Then we talked about how to power up water and food so it always works for your health. Then you just read the steps to evaluate the prescriptions and supplements you are taking or thinking about taking.

I now want to discuss and describe the next step to become more powerfully in charge of your energy field to specifically focus on certain areas of your body. They are called scalar waves.

Dr. Valerie Hunt has been a leader in the scientific world and spent a number of years working in this area of scalar waves. She has coined the word *bioscalar* to refer to scalar energy in living systems. She suggests that in a state of conscious focus, humans can direct positive energy in the form of electromagnetic frequencies from outside the body towards an area of our body that is struggling. The movement of these waves is pulled in straight lines from all different directions towards our body, which is always in the center. Here is a diagram depicting this movement:

Wave # 1----------> (Body) <---------- Wave # 2

I so appreciate Dr. Hunt's description of the powerful abilities we humans naturally have and are capable of working with for our own benefit. All disease within the physical body begins with cells slowing down, becoming sticky, and then clumping together. It is certain emotions that are considered negative such as guilt, regret, shame, and hate that start the process of creating illness. These emotions are dense and vibrate ever so slowly as compared to the emotions of love, caring, and happiness, which vibrate extremely fast. We humans are capable of creating these energetic waves to create illness, but the great news is that we humans have the ability to create our vitality, health, and well-being.

The next diagram shows an image of the entire human body and the correct direction in pulling energy to your body from outside inward in straight lines. It is key to energetically pull straight, direct lines to you from opposite directions. You do this with your thoughts and draw it into your body with your inhalations.

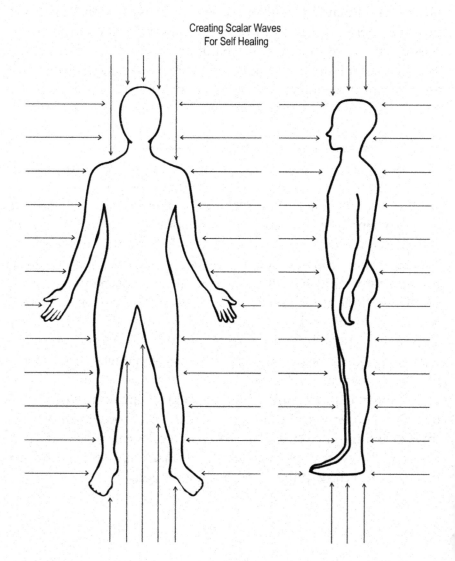

Creating Scalar Waves
For Self Healing

Steps to Create Scalar Waves within Your Physical Body

1. Be playful. Take care to feel your natural empowerment first.

2. Decide the organ or area of your body where you want to direct the healing.

3. Notice the natural rhythm of your breathing . . . then focus on all the sensations of inhaling.

4. Look at the diagram. As you inhale, imagine that you are drawing energy into the center of your body from opposite directions. Imagine drawing in straight lines of energy from two opposite directions into the center of your body at the same time. Begin with inhaling:

5. Front to back and back to front.

6. Then down into your head and up through your feet.

7. Then coming in from the right side of your body and at the same time coming in from the left.

8. Think, imagine, and direct the straight lines of energy coming into the core of your body and into your head and legs.

9. Notice the serene, soothing energy collecting into a quiet pool throughout the center of your body.

10. Once you are filled with a still pool of energy, direct the still pool to go to the exact location that is ill or painful.

11. Be careful when creating commands. Use only the most *positive words describing the results you want*. (Never include any words that describe the negative things happening to you. For example, do not use words such as pain, trauma, disease).

12. Use directives such as: give me peace now, grant me emotional healing now, grant me physical healing now, rebuild tissue now, absorb all growths now.

13. Focus the positive command to the area of your body that needs the healing.

14. Continue your focus for ten minutes at a time.

Summary of Action Steps to Heal and Release

1. Develop a relationship by communicating with your body in general.

2. Develop a relationship by communicating with the illness.

3. Get to know and understand the illness.

4. Water and food are medicines too. Power them up.

5. Assess and evaluate your prescriptions and supplements then talk to your physician.

6. Alter the energy within your body by generating your own scalar waves.

Chapter 18

Cause #3: Your Current Life Traumas and Losses

"Life isn't about waiting for the storms to pass. It is about learning to dance in the rain."
—Vivian Greene, Author of Sparkles and Guns

Let's begin this chapter with a portion of this session. These transcriptions from real sessions describe the profound impact a soul retrieval has for an individual. They describe it better than I could ever do.

TZ: You keep taking classes and videos to learn about intuition and you say you have many sessions with people like me (to teach you how to be intuitive). You want to hear about it, but you do not take action to become an intuitive. Something is not happening for you. Check into it while you are with me so we can get to the bottom of it.

Client: You are right. There is a big block there . . . a bad experience. I feel like I am going to make a mistake and not have good guidance.

TZ: You just called out for a guide (earlier in this session), and you got this old man who looks like a delivery person from the 1940s. You were already suspicious, so you sent out suspicious vibrations and signals outward and you got a suspicious spirit that says it is a guide. I learned the hard way and did not have a teacher. I don't want people to suffer and struggle like I struggled, so that is why I am teaching people to live at this level of awareness.

Client: Well . . . It could be I just do not feel like I am worthy.

TZ: I am hearing that more and more from people. Here is my response. You are sitting here alive with me, and I am alive. Our aliveness is our spirit. That aliveness is what leaves us at the time of death. That aliveness is our spirit. When we do mediumship, that is the aliveness of someone we are perceiving. Spirits are in our yard, in our houses, in our cars, and at work. They are everywhere. It is part of the continuum of the universe. You keep having sessions and classes with teachers like me, trying to become more intuitive. But your unworthiness stops you from putting it into action. Would you call out this command right now?

Client: Yes.

TZ: *Divine and sacred specialty guide, tell me right now the exact cause of my unworthiness!* Then pause and see what jumps into your awareness.

Client: (Long pause) My mother. I am 3 years old. I am nothing to her. I was so miserable. My guide says that I am not unworthy, you just think that you are. My mom could not handle being a mother . . . very abusive. She had three children in a very short time.

TZ: My guides are saying that you believed her, and you swallowed your mother's crap. You have already told me you have physical trouble in your stomach. It is because you swallowed your mother's crap.

Client: I am amazed that she did not kill one of us.

TZ: See what pops in when I ask you this question. Always take the pop because it will be the clearest information. What beliefs did you swallow from your mother and make your own?

Client: I am not worth anything. I am a mistake. I do not trust. Never look bad or make a mistake. I am a misfit. We kids made her life so unhappy. We were responsible for her misery.

TZ: If you keep doing this the way that you are doing this, you are always making your mother more important than you are. You have been trained by an expert to be unworthy. I am saying some tough things to you here.

Client: Then there are still a lot of energetic signatures that I am not aware.

TZ: Yes! Most people just put Band-Aides on their troubles or like peeling the layers off the onion. I want to go to the exact point of origin causing the struggle. Now tell me this. Go back to your three-year-old self right now and see where you find her. It will feel like you are just making it up but let it unfold like a movie.

Client: She is in the kitchen. When Mom gets out of control she is just not there. I am kneeling next to her. She is up by the ceiling.

TZ: I want you to focus on your little girl and not focus on your mother. Make sure the three-year-old knows that you are there with her.

Client: She knows because I put my hands on her to ground her.

TZ: Let her look at you and you look at her. Focus on each other and not your Mother. I want you two to do this together. Get all of the negative out of your little one and also out of you. Take out all the trauma, all the guck, all the old stuff out of your physical bodies and give it back to her. Help your little three-year-old because she is so young. Now this is important: It does not matter what your mother does with it. Just give it back to her no matter what. I will be quiet until you speak.

Client: (Long pause of quiet) I can feel almost all of it gone but there is still black around my feet and around my three-year-old's heart and chest.

TZ: She needs some help. So you get in charge and pull the black out of your little one and give it back and make sure you get it all.

Client: There are so many tendrils everywhere . . . They are not black anymore.

TZ: I am telling you they should not be there. Get in charge of you and your little one. Pull them out at the root from both of you. Make sure you get it all.

Client: There is still something not right about my three-year-old's brain. Tendrils are tangled up in a mass and do not want to come out. It is difficult to pull them out. It is not easy.

TZ: Then you need to guide your little one to help in her own process. She needs to push it all out of her head as you also pull it out. Do this completely together.

Client: Okay.

TZ: Now we have a couple more steps to do. Ask for the most perfect cleansing filter to be there for you right now and see what appears for you.

Client: It is moving and undulating like silver threads sitting in a platinum gel.

TZ: Now make sure that your little one does this together with you. You and your little one, take back every single thing that your mother took from both of you and everything that you lost to her. Take back your confidence, your power, your happiness, your worthiness, and bring it back through this filter so it is all cleaned off . . . Just the pure you comes back and place it into your younger self and your current self right now. And make sure you get all of it. Place it all back inside both of you.

Client: (Very long pause) All right, we are done.

TZ: Now ask your younger self to release that moment and to come forward with you and mature with you, then merge within you.

Client: We left the house and went down the sidewalk, and we both got older together. It feels really different. It is almost like I feel vibrancy in my blood.

TZ: Yes, this is very real, and you truly just did that. Notice the assimilation now and over the next few days. You might write things down as you notice things. You feel this physically because you just went back (in time) and went through this profound healing and then brought her back to you. You need to go look into the mirror to see the difference in your face.

Client: It's like putting on a new energetic dress . . .

Painful Memories, Soul Fragments, and Disassociation

When I ask you this question, notice what leaps into your mind. Do you have a painful memory that keeps rising up in your awareness and the memory still seems so alive or even raw, as if it happened recently? The emotion and the pain might seem a bit haunting sometimes . . . poking at you as if you are reliving it over and over again. What popped into your mind?

Traumatic memories that feel painfully alive, no matter how long ago it happened, is a primary signal that a fragment of you has remained behind in that moment. That explains why it feels so alive even after years or decades have gone by. Notice that the underlying cause is an alarming event in your life and the emotional impact it had on you. It is alive because at some level you are reliving it again and again. That piece is not separate from your soul energy. It is more like a fragment of your energy field became attached or frozen in the trauma of the moment. The rest of your soul's essence stretched on beyond that moment and continued forward in life. Does that make sense?

I have also witnessed what most mental health therapists would diagnose as post-traumatic stress disorder or disassociation. On an energetic level, this appears to the intuitive as an exact shadow of the person. Their shadow can appear just outside of the person's skin and usually off to one side. I have seen it out of the physical body by a few inches to completely standing away from the physical body by twelve inches or more. It looks as if the person has been hit so hard that the soul is knocked off center of the body.

Shamans and indigenous healers have been accomplishing soul retrievals for centuries because they naturally understood that heartache, shock, or trauma grabs hold of a segment of our soul and glues it within a very precise moment in time. Shamans and indigenous healers will go back and collect the soul fragment for the client and bring it to the current client and literally place it into the person's physical body. The shaman then shares what they perceived and how they brought the fragment back to the person and placed it inside of them.

I want to make a clear distinction at this point. The process that I am teaching here has one essential difference from the shamanic method. My goal is to always empower the client, and to do that, I engage the client in their own healing process. To engage you in your own healing I only suggest the next step and then the next step in all healing processes. You actually accomplish healing the fragment of yourself on your own. You then direct the fragment of your younger self to release that moment because it is now completely and permanently healed. You then guide the fragment to come forward to assimilate into your current self and your current body.

Notice in this session that the client did the steps for a soul retrieval on her own and then reported the details with me. I only described the steps to take. She successfully healed a traumatic memory on her own. And so can you.

Client: My homework assignment from the last time we talked was to meet some of my guides. I met four of them. Two of them stepped aside and two of them were to help me with my soul retrieval. I reached out to my guides, and they were very clear about who was to do what. We journeyed together, and my nine-year-old self acknowledged I was there and she knew who I was. But she did not want to have anything to do with us (client and the guide). So, I explained to her that we are now fifty-five years old and I have gone on and lived a full and happy life. I knew she was there on the street corner, and I knew she needed to come home. So she put her guard down a little, but she was refusing to leave that street corner. So I asked her why? She said, *If I leave the corner, I will never see my dad again.*

That never occurred to me in a million years because I knew I saw my dad again because I am now fifty-five years old. It struck me in that moment. I knew she was stuck at nine years old and I knew in my heart and soul that she was still nine years old. She lived in fear every day that she would never see her father again and that was the trauma. I did not realize that because I have moved on from that moment.

So we talked a lot about it. I told her she definitely saw her dad again. I said, "Let me share with you what that was like." We just kept chatting. It was pretty amazing, and it took about two hours. We talked a lot about the next fifty years. She was still sitting on that cement corner. She turned around and I reached out to her. She took my hand and she came home (merged into the client's current physical body). She is here now and always will be here. She is no longer afraid because I shared the memories. When she came home, she can feel the memories.

I am telling you, that little thing is defiant. I have been feeling like, "You can't tell me what to do!" She is no longer on the corner, so I am sort of talking to myself now. I do not think she is 100 percent integrated yet.

TZ: If she was integrated with the current you 100 percent, it would not seem like you were still talking to her. It would feel more like you are talking to yourself. The full assimilation (in a soul retrieval) often takes a full seven days. Just talk to her some more and give her some direction.

Client: I have not been talking to her because I have just been embracing her.

TZ: Just give her some more information while you are embracing her. Tell her, "You are almost complete. We are assimilating and becoming one. Just relax into it. We are the same." Tell her things like that.

Client: She initially was not budging. She was so angry and saying, "Don't tell me what to do!" She was so hurt and angry that she was just stuck there (on that street corner).

TZ: My guides say a different word. She was determined.

Client: She was defiant and determined. "I am not leaving this spot until my dad comes." I told her that he is not coming. I did explain to her that it took many years to understand that it was not because Dad didn't love us. He didn't come back because he did love us. He didn't want us to see the fights and the arguments or something really bad might happen. He was really protecting us. That mellowed her too. That realization helped her as much as anything. But now she is home in all her glory and all her energy!

This is an element (soul fragment) I should have had a long time ago. There were times when I should have said no. It feels like I am home again. Like I have all the tools I needed but didn't have. There has been healing on both sides of us for sure. Then together we went and got our fourteen-year-old. The fourteen-year-old said, "Okay, I've been waiting. I knew I could not come until the nine-year-old came." They both came back to me on the same day.

I want to share with you one more soul retrieval experience.

TZ: What is going on about your belief that you are a powerful link in the system?

What happened in your life around five years old?

Client: That's when the abuse heightened.

TZ: It stands out in your field very strongly. You are still carrying a sense of victim in your energy field.

Client: I have already done a lot of work around this issue. I feel helpless. I took care of my younger brother when our mother passed. So I always feel like I will take it on for him so he does not suffer. I always have this "Mom energy." I will take it on for you so you do not hurt.

TZ: I know that you realize this does not help your brother either.

Client: Yes, I realize that. I do it with everyone. How do I change this pattern?

TZ: Would you be willing to do a healing with me? Take what pops when I ask you this. What is your most painful moment that keeps rising up and stays in your memories?

Client: Around 8 years old I went to my mother and told her that her brother is hurting me. My mother's sister was there as well. My aunt said, "Don't believe her. She is lying and not telling the truth." Something happened to me around that age that I decided it is not safe to speak my truth. I remember everything about that moment. I remember the room. My mother told me not to lie and off she sent me. That is what is coming up for me.

TZ: You describe this memory so clearly. I want you to imagine stretching yourself outward and go back to be with your little one in that moment. How do you know that she realizes you are there for her?

Client: She is smiling at me.

TZ: Good. Now I want you to call out to your divine and sacred healers to be there for both of you. Tell them to help you take all of that pain out of you, all of your loss of power and loss of your voice, and give it back to both your mother and your aunt. Take your time and make sure that you get it all out of both of you.

Client: All kinds of things are coming out of us.

TZ: Get it all out of both of you and give it back to who and where it came from.

Client: A lot of it is in my heart.

TZ: Make sure you get it all. Help your younger self and ask her to help too. She needs to know that she has the power to remove it as well.

Client: (coughing) I saw a wire going all through my jaw.

TZ: Get it out of you and give it back. It now feels more complete. Now ask your specialist to create the most beautiful and effective filter for both of you.

Client: I saw a sucking tube, sucking things up just like at a bank drive up.

TZ: Now I want you to take back everything that was taken from you and everything that you gave away to your mother and your aunt. Bring it through the filter all cleaned off and put it inside of you and your younger self.

Client: Interesting. I took out shame and lack of integrity. My voice, trust, power, and my self-belief. Joy and playfulness came back. Joy and trust came back. It was an image or an object. A sword came out of my throat.

TZ: Now ask your younger self if there is anything else she wants or needs to happen?

Client: Hmm. She says to be fully integrated.

TZ: That is exactly the next step to take in this healing. Ask her if she is willing to completely release this moment and move forward toward you and mature and merge with you right now in this moment.

Client: That was weird. I saw an image like paper dolls. All that coming in together and then she was growing through me and inside of me.

TZ: My guides are saying that they want you to notice the assimilation over the next four days. In four days, you will notice more and more. This was very real, and this is a soul retrieval. It is about engaging you with your younger self in this healing. It is similar to the Native American soul retrieval but with differences.

Client: Look at the card (tarot card) that I selected today! It is called White Eagle. (Client holds up a card with a Native American male in full headdress to show me). It says, "Connect to your lineage. A family wound or pattern can be healed now. I am understanding my situation with my brother more clearly now too. You just cannot make this stuff up!

TZ: This is only the beginning. This has not even fully assimilated yet. You truly went back in time for the healing of that moment that was so painful, and you truly connected with your younger self and you truly brought that piece of yourself back.

Two Methods to Heal and Forever Release Trauma

All three clients gave me permission to share their stories to help you heal the ways they have. I sincerely want you to realize that my part in these soul retrievals was very minor. I only mentioned each next step in this healing process. Every single client I have ever worked with has completely accomplished their soul retrieval on their own, and so can you.

When something in your past feels raw, it only means that you have literally left a piece of yourself behind in that trauma. From now on, do not push aside any memories. When the memory rises up it is intuitively sending its message to you. The message is telling you that it is time to heal. It is not telling you that it is time to suffer again and again, but that is what most people do with memories of trauma.

Hear me say this to you now. You do not need to remember or relive the ordeal, or know all the details of the distress, to heal and release it. In these steps the energy healing will go where it needs to go. You do not have to remember an experience, or know the details, to completely and permanently heal it. This is vitally important and so I will repeat it again:

Important: You do not have to remember an experience, or know the details, to completely and permanently heal it.
Any trauma that happens has happened in your past. It does not matter if the past was an hour ago or twenty years ago or even longer than that. You do not need to remember the past moments or even know the details to permanently heal and completely release it. If you were mistreated in any way as a child or as an adult it is now time to take your power back. Do a soul retrieval just for you for every moment and every memory that feels raw and pokes at your heart. If you have any memories that keep coming up, it's time to heal every single moment and to take your power back. Follow these exact steps in the exact order that they are stated here. Read it through a couple of times to get the feel of them. Then take action for yourself:

Soul Retrieval Steps

1. Remember that intuitive information and intuitive energy work will always *feel* like your imagination, but it is real, and it is truly happening. It will become like a movie in your mind. Just let it unfold.

2. Stretch out and send the current 'you' back to wherever you find your younger self. Find the younger you just minutes before the incident happens.

3. Make sure the younger self knows you are there. How does the younger you know you are there now?

4. Take all the terrible energy out of both of you and give it back to the wrongdoer or to the traumatic moment. Notice what the energy looks like as you remove it from both of you.

5. Scan each other to make sure you got it all. Look everywhere to make sure you have left nothing behind. Look around your heart and any injured areas. Get it all out.

6. Give absolutely all of the energy back to the wrongdoer or to the moment. **Important: It does not matter what the wrongdoer does with it. Just give it back.**

7. Call out to a divine and sacred guide who specializes in powerful cleansing filters. Command that a filter be created for you. Watch it appear and how beautiful it is.

8. Now take back all that was taken from you and all that you gave away. Bring all of you through the filter so only the purest 'you' comes back to you. Place all of the purest 'you' back into you and your younger self. Make sure you get it all.

9. Take a moment to sense the complete wholeness of who you are. Feel your new empowerment.

10. Now with all your empowerment stare the wrongdoer directly in the eyes until they change in some way. Hold your look until they change.

11. Tell your younger self to feel the complete healing of that moment.

12. Tell your younger self to permanently release that moment, come forward with you, mature, and then merge together with you.

13. Notice delightful changes over the next three to seven days as your younger self assimilates within you.

Over many years I have discovered that there are two phenomenal healing methods to permanently heal but also forever release heartache and trauma. We just examined the beautiful healing method of soul retrievals. There is another healing method that is excellent for painful or traumatic moments in your past. This method was developed by a man named Raymon Grace. I love this man! He is down to earth and gets to the point. He is also a masterful healer, so I give him all the credit for his three-step healing technique. Since he is a dowser, he uses a pendulum with each step. A pendulum is not necessary if you do not have one or do not have any training in how to use it. If you do not use a pendulum, I ask that you allow yourself to sense, feel, or see the activity that is happening. Just like the soul retrieval, these steps are real and the healing is actually happening.

I will tell you one of my very personal stories about healing an old painful trauma in my life with these steps.

At the time, I had been divorced from my husband for twenty-five years. Together we have two children and now five grandchildren. We often found ourselves together in the same room for birthdays and family events. Every time we were together, I would walk up to him and say, "Hi!" to that man. For twenty-five years he would turn his face away from me and act like I did not exist and did not just greet him. For twenty-five years I repeated my same greeting just to see what would happen but each time he turned away. But do you know what else was happening? I noticed that, occasionally, painful moments would pop up out of nowhere and I would see our fights and hear his terrible words in my memories.

One day my guides got through to me and I heard, "You have been healing others for years. Why aren't you healing yourself and these moments of heartache?" That stopped me in my tracks. Good heavens, I need to heal my traumatic past too. I immediately took action and did Raymon's three steps for the most pain-filled memory that kept poking at me over the years. I felt the complete release and knew it was over. Surprise! All the other painful memories began to rise up in my memories, so I repeated the steps over and over for each memory. This went on for at least three weeks and then the memories stopped.

Soon after doing my last healing sessions, my ex-husband and I found ourselves together in my daughter's home for a grandchild's birthday party. I did what I always have done for twenty-five years. I walked up to that man and said, "Hi!" He turned, looked up into my eyes and said, "Hi Tina."

Now here is an important point that needs to be discussed in a very clear way. I did not include my ex-husband in my three step healing sessions. I did not include him because he did not give me permission. Only do healing work with other people if they give you permission. You can ask for permission by calling the other person on the phone or you can ask the person intuitively. To intuitively ask someone for permission, you picture them in your mind's eye, say their full name when you ask them for permission. This communication is a telepathic interchange. If the other person sends you a telepathic refusal you might perceive it in different ways. The person might frown at you. They might turn away from you, or the word "no" leaps into your mind. You might feel a downward sinking sensation. A "yes" might come as a smile, a "yes" popping into your mind, or an uplifting sensation. If you get a "no," it is vital that you honor the "no."

My ex-husband did not give me permission when I intuitively asked him. I didn't know what to do, so I asked my guides. They said, "Do not send the healing to your ex-husband. Send it to each painful moment and not to the other person." I want to emphasize two important guidelines to you:

1. Never send energy work to another person unless they give you permission. Without permission, you could be slipping into a darker form of energy work by making someone do something that you want and not necessarily what they want.

2. If other people are part of your traumatic memories then direct these healings steps to the exact moment.

Guidelines to Raymon Grace's Three-Step Process to Heal and Release Trauma

- Do the three steps all in one sitting. You can do as many sittings as it takes until you feel or sense a difference in some way. Most people, including me, describe it as a sense of relief when the healings are finished.

- You do not need to know all the details of the past event. Direct it to all of the causes.

- You can use a pendulum for each step or not. If you do not use a pendulum, just stay with each step until you sense the action of each step subsiding on its own.

- The first step of the command is to scramble. Simply imagine that the motion and action is like scrambling eggs. You are actually breaking up the density of the event.

- When you command to neutralize in the second step, you will feel all the emotions drain out of the past traumatic experience. You are actually removing all emotions from the event.

- The third step requires special attention. You must use the exact words that describe what you want the old traumatic times to be transformed into. A useful guideline is to use precise, exact, clear words that are the opposite of how you have been suffering. For example, if your traumatic past experience left you depressed and hopeless then you will want it transformed into joy and powerfully confident. If the trauma left you afraid of people then you might want it transformed into bravery with other people.

- Read the steps first and rewrite them on an index card or paper and fill in the blanks with the precise words that clearly define what you want scrambled and neutralized and then the exact words describing the positive results you want.

- Use the exact same words in the scramble step and the neutralize step.

- Use the words that describe your goals in the transformation step.

The Three Steps

Call out to your most powerful divine and sacred specialty healing guides, then command the following in these exact words:

Step 1: *Now completely and permanently scramble the exact point of origin when* (name the event) *happened to me,* (your name).

Step 2: *Now completely and permanently neutralize the exact point of origin when* (name the event) *happened to me,* (your name).

Step 3: *Now completely and permanently transform all that has been scrambled and neutralized into* (name the exact positive words that describe what you want), *now!*

Summary of Action Steps to Heal and Release

1. Allow yourself to truly notice each raw, painful memory that rises up.

2. Know now that memories are signals that it is time to take action and heal.

3. You are your own healer. I only give you the steps to take. You are the one doing the steps.

4. Do a soul retrieval for every painful memory.

5. Do the three-step healing method.

Chapter 19

Cause #4: Your Relationships

"A relationship should never take anything away.
It should give to you."

—Janie Kaminer

Yes, relationships are one of the causes of illness. Check yourself to see if this is a new idea for you. This book is about you, not everyone that you love or worry about. You do not need to be more important than everyone else. Your goal is to be equally important, not more important. Get in charge of yourself first in order to achieve the healthier you. Your enriched energy and awareness will naturally expand outward to others. Your health is the greatest healing you can give to the ones you care about most. As a registered nurse with a board specialty certification in mental health and as a Gestalt trained mental health counselor, I could go hundreds of directions regarding relationships. But I've decided to discuss the concerns and problems that I hear the most from my clients over the years. To summarize the primary problem that people describe in their sessions is this:

In relationships, no one thinks anyone is doing anything right, and you want everyone to change and do it right, but no one changes the way you want them to change.

Most misery that I consistently see in my practice is a client desperately wanting, trying, and hoping their cherished loved one's thoughts, beliefs, and behavior change. This is the dilemma that causes stress and sometimes unbearable heartache for so many people in their relationship problems. There are a few other issues, but this one is consistent. Notice yourself now for a moment. What words or actions do you use when you try to get a certain thing to happen? Are you trying to get something or someone to change? Are you trying to fix something or someone? Are you trying to help or to change a family member? As a mental health counselor for over thirty-five years now I consistently see this struggle in every type of relationship that exists.

First of all, each person is such a unique individual living a unique life with unique experiences. No one else is like you so no one else can think the way you do, make decisions the way you do, and live the life that you do. As you keep trying to get someone to change toward what you think is for the better, your own stresses and internal conflicts continue to build. Your own happiness and your health slips away, sometimes slowly and sometimes fast.

Constantly and consistently take the stance to be a fascinated scientific observer of every single person's actions and the words that they say or do. Each human is an eternal struggling soul trying to make it through life. Observe and learn about each person as a struggling soul. Notice without judgment because a scientist does not judge. The clearest intuitive observes, explores, and tries to learn from each situation.

This client has focused on her parents for so much of her life.

Client: When you guided me through the healing steps (soul retrieval) and told me it would take seven days, I thought you meant it would heal the relationship between my parents and me. It did not change them, but it was not about them! Now I am not bothered by them and they do not have power over me anymore. The healing wasn't that I am going to have a wonderful relationship with my parents. This was the healing. So, thank you!

TZ: Well, you are welcome. Let me say this in greater detail. The seven-day time period was the time my guides said that your younger self and your current self would need to assimilate together. That healing was about your younger self coming back into you all cleaned off and pure. It was not about your parents changing because they probably won't. It is you that have changed!

Client: (giggles) I feel more whole. Now when I wake up in the night, I am calling myself back from other moments with my parents and from my team leader at my work and from other people. Most of the time I am giving away my power and they are not taking it from me. It was taken from me as a child, but not anymore! I am now in an observer position where I feel all versions of my five-year-old self and all other versions of myself have come together. We are not the victim and we are not the powerful one. We are all on one team. I am becoming more of the observer of things around me. My husband is noticing such changes with me.

TZ: This is just beautiful and amazing. I want you to become a fascinated observer of life around you.

The more you allow yourself to advance your personal level of intuitive awareness, the more you will understand others. You will judge and criticize less. You will expand to see the world from a broader perspective. You will see yourself and others more as a soul on a long, long journey filled with learning. You will also realize and know things about people around you because you are more intuitive and living at a more intuitive level.

Amy Jo Ellis works with the Full Court of Atonement, which includes numerous highly evolved spirit guides for issues you are asking to be resolved. Atonement is about bringing peace, resolution, or settlement among each other. I have worked with the Full Court of Atonement for a long time now to resolve an issue with a neighbor, or I have placed myself into the Court for many disputes or concerns with family, co-workers, and others over the years as well.

In my experience the officials sitting on the Courts change with each issue or situation that you ask for assistance. My sense is that the divine officials are specialists, and those specialists change depending on the people or the issue. **Important: Do not try to use the Full Court of Atonement to try to make someone do what you want them to do.**

Here is a quote from Amy Jo Ellis, which is a command for the Full Court of Atonement. This one touches my heart every time I work with it. Please consider using it:

> *"I, (your full name) apologize to myself for holding my heart hostage by demanding that things be different than how they turned out. I apologize to my heart for hurting myself daily, telling myself that I needed someone else to change instead of changing what I could control, which is my own ability to choose to be whole, happy, and complete with things exactly as they are meant to be. If they were meant to be different . . . they would already be different. I ask to look back over my timeline and to call Full Courts of Atonement on all areas in my life where I took my happiness hostage and tried to ransom myself to force others to change. I ask for all this energy to be corrected on the astral plane."*

I want to offer you a flexible framework for commanding the Full Court of Atonement for your personal issues. Again, your wording is the most valuable factor in any command and that still applies to the Full Court of Atonement:

I ask that I, your full name, full names of all others involved, all be placed into the Full Court of Atonement in order to resolve and clear all conflicts and transforming it into complete understanding, complete appreciation and complete unconditional love in our relationships with each other on all dimensions and all timeframes. So Be It . . .

How did Everyone Become More Important than You?

Remember one of the eleven keys to constantly do for yourself is: Save Yourself First. We humans so readily make someone else more important than we are. How did someone else become more important than you? How did that happen in the first place? It happens over the years and it happens little by little. People can become so focused on family members or friends that they know very little about themselves. I have had hour-long counseling sessions with clients who do not speak about themself at all even when I ask a personal question. It is as if they are not in their own life. Life is outside of them. It is external all around them.

People lose themselves in the disarray of others around them. They have very little knowledge about themselves. They worry and agonize about individuals in their family and cannot describe themselves for even a few minutes. Everyone around them is dramatically important.

My client was a highly recognized individual sports coach for highly recognized athletes. At the peak of her career, she quit her position and moved across the country to take care of her father. She finally told me that her father stayed in his bedroom and rarely knew who she was. Now, there could have been other factors causing her to make that decision, but what kept coming up in counseling was the fact that she did not feel important in her own life. She quickly lost her empowerment, her physical strength, and her confidence.

Now what about you? Have you stopped living your life, or a great part of your life, for someone else? Notice what pops into your awareness. Take these steps first to learn more about you and your relationships:

1. Imagine standing over at the outer edge of your life.

2. Observe like the most fascinated scientist and notice everything.

3. Notice:

    • What does your life look like in general?

    • Who stands out as the most important, then second, then third? Where are you located on the list of important people?

- What was the exact moment that you lost track of 'you'?

4. Decide if you want to change anything. You are in charge of every second of your life. It really is up to you.

5. Call out for a divine and sacred guide who specializes in helping you create your best life. Notice who arrives and ask many questions such as:

- What is important for me to realize first about my life?

- Am I struggling to deserve a different life?

- What is the first small step to take to live more in my own life?

6. If you decide to put 'you' back into your life, make the first step extremely small. It has to be a doable step that you can actually accomplish.

7. Work with this guide all day, every day. Communicate and communicate some more.

Your Negative Patterns that Keep Repeating

We all have patterns in our life that keep repeating. What patterns do you keep finding yourself in? What situations and with what type of people do you keep finding yourself in the middle of . . . again? Stop here and notice your patterns . . .

My real-life example kept happening when I worked in upper management for home healthcare companies. I always found myself deep in conflict and mismanagement. Four different companies were sold, and four different times the new owners came in and fired all the administrators and regional managers to place their own people in those positions. Once I was fired the day before Thanksgiving.

After the fourth time of buy-outs and mass firings of management, it occurred to me that there was an unbelievable, intense pattern that kept playing out in my life. I stopped and finally asked spirit, "What am I to learn and understand from this pattern?" After my guides stopped dancing around in laughter they said, "You are not meant to work for other companies, and you are not meant to do home healthcare! You are supposed to work for yourself and counsel people." When I received that message it suddenly seemed so obvious that I was embarrassed. My embarrassment made the guides laugh even more until I laughed with them.

A repetitive pattern is a glaring message that you are not learning what you must learn to continue forward in your development. When you finally notice that your patterns keep repeating in your life, you too will be amazed. Life patterns come in all shapes and forms, often involving relationships, work, locations, business, money, love, battles, accidents . . . there is no end to the powerful repetitive messages that signal a change is required. Examine your negative patterns now. Ask your divine and sacred guides this two-step command:

Tell me or show me, your full name, *exactly what I am to learn now from this pattern of* _____ *repeating again in my life.* (Pause and take the pop of wisdom.)

Show me, your full name, *the exact steps to alter, heal, and release all negative patterns in my life now.*

Who Is Your Greatest Teacher?

Who in your life consistently causes you the most pain, the most sorrow, the most agitation or anger, or is a constant thorn in your side? That person is your greatest teacher. They have taken on a difficult role for themselves but also for you as well. When someone in your life plays out the role of a powerful life teacher, you cannot ignore it. Each painful interaction is another prospect, another chance to learn about you. It appears that they are the issue, but they are not the issue. It is not about learning more about your greatest teacher or trying to change them. They carry a position and act out the role to goad and prod you into change or awareness of some sort. You make the choice to react in a negative way or take a different action in a positive way.

If you keep focusing on and analyzing that person, you will never resolve the conflict and discord. This person, who consistently creates deep emotions within you, will continue to draw your attention until there is a change within you. You must learn more about yourself, not more about your nemesis. Stop judging, crying, lamenting over this person. Turn around and look into your own eyes. Look into your soul and find your next step, to discover a depth of wisdom inside of you that you have never reached before.

Negative People Cording into You

Negative people are not the only ones who create negative energetic cords. You can inadvertently create negative cords to another individual without deliberately meaning to do so. Thoughts focused on a person that are filled with emotion can possibly create an energetic connection with them. It is up to you if that is a positive or a negative connection. For example, if you feel intense emotions such as jealousy, shock, fury, devastation, offense, rage, or shattering disappointment, those emotions literally jet out from you and focus on the other person. That in itself creates a thick, dense cord that appears muddy, cloudy, in dark brown or gray. In the same way someone who feels powerful negative emotions about you can inadvertently or deliberately lash out at you and form a negative cord into you.

When we humans care deeply about a person, beautiful, thin, light, shimmery, cordlike energy forms between the two of you. People who feel positive about you will have positive cording connections with you. In my experience I have never found any reason to disconnect a positive cord between those we love and those who love us in return.

When you scan yourself and become aware of a dim or even dark-colored cord connected to you anywhere in your body or your energy field, you must first, honestly, and without judgment, question who created the negative cord? Does it flow out of you, or does it flow from somewhere outside of you and go into your energy field or your physical body? If it flows at you and into you, then follow it along to see who is at the other end. You might be surprised at who is on the other end of it, or you might already know who sent it. Remember:

- You are no longer a victim.
- You are in charge of you, so take charge.
- Never cut a cord because that does not heal the situation.

Two Methods to Heal Relationships

1. **Steps to Remove and Heal Negative Cords**
    - You have discovered a dim, dark cord somewhere in your energy field or within your physical body.
    - Notice the direction that it seems to flow. Follow the cord to the end to sense or see who is there.
    - Command: *Divine and sacred guides who specialize in removing negative cords, completely and permanently pull out and remove all tendrils and all particles of all negative cords from my body and energy field now. Give back the cords and give back all the negativity to the sender now. It is theirs and not mine.*
    - At the same time, you take charge of 'you' and take action to assist the specialists to release and remove the cord.
    - When it is gone you then command the healers: *Completely and permanently fill every single space and place where the negative cord used to be with vitality, Light of Source and unconditional love now.*

2. **Three Step Healing for Relationships**

Here again are the guidelines for the Raymon Grace three step healing method:

- Do the three steps all in one sitting. You can do as many

sittings as it takes until you feel or sense a difference in some way. Most people, including me, describe it as a sense of relief when the healings are finished. You do not need to know all the details of the past event. Direct it to the causes.

- You can use a pendulum for each step or not. If you do not use a pendulum just stay with each step until you sense the action of each step subsiding on its own.

- The first step of the command is to scramble. Simply imagine the motion and action is like scrambling eggs. You are actually breaking up the density of the event.

- When you command to neutralize in the second step, you will feel all the emotions drain out of the negative relationship. Neutralizing actually means removing all negative emotions from the relationship.

- The third step requires special attention. You must use the exact words that describe what you want the negative relationship to be transformed into. A useful guideline is to use clear, precise, exact words that are the opposite of how you have been suffering. For example, if this relationship is about fighting constantly, then you might want it transformed into unconditional love, understanding, peace. If the relationship leaves you fearing for your life, then you want it transformed into: Stop now, permanent end of all connections with (name the person).

- Read the steps first and rewrite them on an index card or paper and fill in the blanks with the precise words that clearly define what you want scrambled and neutralized and then the exact words describing the positive results you want.

- Use the exact same words in the scramble step and the neutralize step.

- Use the words that describe your goals in the transformation step.

You just read some basic guidelines. Invite in your most powerful divine and sacred healers, then command the following in these exact words:

- Step 1: *Now completely and permanently scramble the exact points of origin causing the current negative relationship with my* state type of relationship (e.g. son, wife, friend), full name of person.

- Step 2: *Now completely and permanently neutralize the exact points of origin causing the current negative relationship with my* state type of relationship (e.g. son, wife, friend), full name of person.

- Step 3: *Now completely and permanently transmute and transform all that has been scrambled and neutralized into* (e.g. relief, release, Divine Love, permanent peace, etc.)

Summary of Action Steps to Heal and Release

1. Use the Full Court of Atonement to resolve all types of conflicts and issues between you and others.

2. Each person is a struggling soul on a long journey. Be a fascinated observer of every person's actions and the words they say. Observe without judgment.

3. A repetitive pattern in life is a glaring message that you are to learn the deeper message beneath the pattern.

4. Your greatest teacher in this life will consistently cause you the most pain, the most sorrow, the most agitation or anger. You must learn more about yourself, not more about the teacher.

5. Cutting negative cords is not healing them. They must be removed to heal.

6. You can transform a relationship into the positive.

Chapter 20

Cause #5: Your Environment

"The goal of life is to make your heartbeat match
the beat of the universe, to match your
nature with Nature."
—Joseph Campbell

Your Environment is Negatively Affected by Many Things on Many Levels

This energy worker thought she was about to provide a medical intuitive session focusing on her client's physical body, but when she commanded to be told or shown the cause of her medical conditions, the following instantly happened.

> "I did some work for a lady last week remotely and while tuning into her I was told (by her guides) to look at the land the house is built on. There was a big (energetic) crack in the ground and there was a soldier standing at the end of the crack. So I called on a guide to come forward to help, and I was amazed.
>
> "A pure white, glowing staircase appeared from the crack. All these souls started walking out. He (the soldier) was standing there watching, holding his gun. He was wearing a red tunic with gold buttons, a tall black hat with gold on it, and the gun had like a bell at the end of it. Then the last two

souls came out. They turned around and it looked like they were pulling a rope to bring the steps up. As they pulled the steps up, the crack sealed. They all proceeded to a lovely, arched door that had a baby-blue-coloured light. The soldier then looked back at me and saluted, then he went towards the door.

"I later asked for feedback from the lady, and she said she couldn't believe the difference as it seemed to happen within the hour of me doing it. What an amazing experience! I was going to do a medical intuitive reading with her, and as I said before, you never know where you'll go or what you'll see. A healing took place for many there . . . Still amazes me!"

I began to notice that the environment is occasionally the cause of a medical illness. In the case above, spirit people in the environment were interfering with this client's health. The environment, in turn, was affected by human emotions of spirit people, lingering within the woman's property.

Our environment is not just our home or apartment. It not only includes the structure of the building you live in but also the land it is on. It includes your workplace, your fun place, your journey down the road between one place to another, an intersection, a railroad crossing, or even an airplane. Your environment becomes anywhere you are located at the time. I have driven past auto wrecks and have been negatively affected by it on an emotional level and on a spiritual level at the exact same time. For weeks, the spirit of a young male about seventeen or eighteen years old would appear in the front seat passenger side of my car as I drove home from work. He told me his name was Bobby and he died at the spot where his parents placed the cross. The next day I looked more closely at the cross along the side of the road. This cross marked the exact place where he died in an automobile wreck and, indeed, the name "Bobby" was etched into it. Later that week, I was driving down that same road and I saw a tall, thin male walk across the road at that same spot. When I got to that wide-open place in the road, no one was physically there. Because I have been a medium since I can remember I was not negatively affected by him or that section of the road, but someone who drives through that same area every day might pick up the intense density of emotions that were lingering at the site of that automobile wreck.

Here is one more example of spirit people potentially causing stress or illness in living people through a certain environment. Robert Moss, author of *Sidewalk Oracles*, describes what he saw with his "inner senses" just as he was about to begin teaching his workshop.

> "It was not really a surprise when I noticed through my inner senses that we had been joined by the spirits of several hundred men in blue and gray, soldiers killed on both sides in the American Civil War who had apparently remained close to the place where their bodies had fallen. I requested their senior officers to step forward. I suggested to them that they were welcome to audit our class but that it was primarily intended for the living who had joined our circle and that I would be grateful if they would remain outside our perimeter and maintain good order."

Based on their uniforms, those spirit people have been there for a very long time. I want to point out that, in this example from Robert Moss, those soldiers in battle mode could have been the primary underlying cause of conflict amongst the staff and the attendees at that retreat center. Their presence could keep up an agitated, argumentative feeling to the grounds and the buildings, and no one would ever figure that out unless they lived at an intuitive level of life.

Again, I want to emphasize that it is emotions in the moment that keep the spirit people focused on a certain environment. Those emotions remain and even build over time, and as living people are affected, they too add to the energy of the old conflict of war. Notice how Moss simply discussed things with the leaders in a matter-of-fact dialogue. They seemed to agree. But notice that, at least in his book, he did not do a healing and release for those souls. Communicate in a back-and-forth dialogue in a matter-of-fact manner. Never chase deceased people away! They are real people who need help to heal and release the emotions that locked them to that environment.

Negative thought forms, located in certain environments, are caused by living people as well as dead people. Negative thoughts, over time, will accumulate in certain locations. Every time a living person has a heavy negative thought and its subsequent emotion, the energy of it accumulates over time.

An example of a common physical location causing illness or tensions could be a busy intersection in your city where many deadly wrecks have happened. Many people drive through that same intersection twice a day and worry that they might be next for a wreck. All that continual worry and fear is dense, and each day it builds up a little more all throughout that certain intersection. People are literally driving through dense thought forms and are being affected by it. A thought form is not a spirit or entity of any kind, but it is a gathering of negative energy that is dense and sticky, and people who have similar emotions will tend to add to the thought form, but also, the thought form will pull towards the person, adding to their struggles even more.

The land, water, and the earth in general is obviously affected by living people as well, and as a result the land becomes toxic, and it circles around to create illness of the living people. The natural environment is thought to be the trigger for many allergies. People think their allergies are caused by the environment, that pollens of trees, shrubs, and grass are the physical cause of their allergies when, in fact, my guides keep informing me that beneath all allergies is an emotional cause.

The clearest example I can think of comes from one of my

mentoring clients. She seemed to be allergic to the world around her. When I commanded, *Tell me or show me now the exact point of origin causing all of the allergies negatively affecting Lori,* I instantly perceived her as a small child with the number six hovering over her head. I said, "I see you at the age of six with an older couple who seem like grandparents. They were talking about their allergies. Right then and there you decided that you wanted to have allergies too so you could be just like your grandparents."

Her emotions sent out an empowered request to the Universe. She sent out a message to receive allergies and she created allergies. If we have that much power at the age of six to create an illness, we adults have even more power and wisdom to create our health. Believe it first, then power up! (To heal allergies, refer back to Soul Retrieval Steps).

The entire earth is our environmental home. Hugh Newman, author of *Earth Grids* and speaker on the History Channel, is known for his exploration of the ancient sights and the energy matrix that is associated with the earth. The earth itself is a living entity, and it too is about 70 percent water. Water is readily affected by emotions within the human body but also the body of the earth. The earth, on its own, has its high energy places and its lower energy places. It has its ley lines, energy grids, vortexes, and patterns. We humans also have our own influences on the earth's energy field way. The earth affects us, and we affect it.

Steps to Heal and Release Spirit People from Your Environment

1. Do not chase spirit people away. Help them. They need something.

2. If you do not see them with your eyes open or in your mind's eye, then directly ask your divine and sacred guides if there are deceased people in your environment. If you receive a "yes," then go to the next step.

3. Ask the spirit person questions and pause to receive the answers to pop into your mind such as: *Who are you? Why*

    are you here in (my house, land, workspace, etc.?) Pause for the answers.

4. Then ask: *Do you realize you are dead? Do you realize staying here in this location is not the best place for you?* Pause for the answers.

5. Inform the dead person that you are calling in specialists to assist them into a new and special life.

6. Call in divine and sacred guides who specialize in transitioning the deceased and take them to the highest place for their transformation into Light and Love.

7. If the dead person resists, be firm and consistent. Keep telling them: *This is not the greatest life for you. There is nothing here for you anymore. Feel the love coming from the guides.*

8. When anything is released, it will be filled and replaced with something powerfully positive. Call in the divine and sacred healing specialists and command: *Fill every space and place where that spirit person used to be with Light, Compassion, and Love.*

I want to begin by reminding you that there are specialists in the physical world for everything, and there are specialists in the non-physical world for everything too. Even the Bible says, "As above, so below." Who knew it applied to spirit specialists too?

Steps to Clear Negative Thought Forms from Your Environment

1. This is like giving your environment a good, long shower.

2. Call out to divine and sacred guides who specialize in removing and cleansing all types of negativity.

3. Command the following: *Now completely and permanently remove all accumulations of negativity on all levels and in all places associated with me,* (your full name).

4. Then command the following: *Now cleanse all spaces and places where the negative used to be with precious, pure, clean*

energy. Permanently place it within, throughout, and around on all levels and in all dimensions."

Steps to Clear Physical Toxins from Your Environment

Raymon Grace is very well known for using these steps to clean up and heal schools for children and for clearing toxins from water and land. Three Step Healing Commands:

Invite in your most powerful divine and sacred healers, then command the following in these exact words:

Step 1: *Now completely and permanently scramble all the exact points of origin causing the toxic, contaminated* (name the land, water, or area, etc.) *at* (name the exact address or location).

Step 2: *Now completely and permanently neutralize all the exact points of origin causing the toxic, contaminated* (name the land, water, or area, etc.) *at* (name the exact address or location).

Step 3: *Now completely and permanently transform all that has been scrambled and neutralized into* (clean, wholesome, vitally alive, etc.) (name the land, water, or area, etc.) *at* (name the exact address or location).

Summary of Action Steps to Heal and Release

1. Here is your playful homework assignment. I ask that you examine your intuitive pops and awareness of different environments. I ask that you notice the gas stations that you always go to, but also the ones you always drive past. Check out your intuitive sensations and awareness about each one. There is more going on than you think. It is not just visual information like one gas station has been recently painted and looks better. What are you truly realizing about these gas stations on a deeper level? Why do you pick the one you usually pick?

2. Practice clearing any type of negativity from your own home, land, and buildings.

3. Clear any and all physical toxins from your personal environment.

4. Talk to deceased people like they are real and need some help, because they are real and need some help, or they would not be bothering you.

Chapter 21

Cause #6: Your Past Life Traumas and Losses

"The vision may be the destination but the journey
began with a past which will stay connected
whatever the sages may say against it—
there is always a hyperlink."

—Amit Abraham

Have you heard the old saying, "Time will heal"? Well, in some cases, time does diminish the sharpness, the viciousness of a painful event, but time does not actually heal the trauma. We are eternal just as the universe is eternal. So, in the realms of eternity this life is merely a swift twinkle and then we are on to other things.

A past life trauma is basically no different from a current life trauma. Both traumas, past life or your current life, can still negatively affect you. It simply does not matter if the trauma seemed to happen three centuries ago or three decades ago. What does matter is the extreme emotions that happened in those experiences. Consider this: both experiences happened in your past and both involved distress and pain, and both profoundly damaged you in some way. The trauma emotionally impacted you. Extreme intense emotions from your current life and extreme intense emotions from your past life can carry forward and continue to interfere in your current experiences today.

Over the years, strange images or stories emerge within people's awareness. These stories rise up in people who do not even believe in past lives. Even now, if you are wondering about past lives or not sure if that can happen, I want you to consider this. If it is not a past life memory to you, then consider it a strange dreamlike experience that still offers you accurate information, but that information is coming to you in story form. Accept it as signals, messages, and crucial information about you and the issues that need to be healed. Believe it as a symbolic story if you do not believe in past lives. It will still allow profound healings and release from your old issues.

The past life experiences in the following sessions speak volumes about past lives causing challenges, struggles, and illnesses in each person's current life.

I want you to notice that I only offer steps to take, and every individual takes the action and receives the information and the healings. So pay attention to the steps along the way.

Client: I really want to learn how to communicate with my own masters for my own healing. I want to talk to them about my own conditions. I am already good with my guides when I am assisting others, but to work on myself, it seems different.

TZ: Now, really think about this. How is it different for you when you work on other people?

Client: When I am helping other people I do not question myself, but when I do this for myself I always question myself. I can concentrate better when I am doing intuitive work for others but not when I am doing this for myself. I doubt myself. I wonder, is this my thinking or is it them (guides)? I have taken intuitive mediumship classes, and I am pretty good for others. I am trying to help myself over all these years, but I still have my problems. Maybe I am not good for myself

TZ: Here is what I just heard you say. You ask your guides and get a response, but you then ask yourself a lot of questions. Do you have a divine specialty guide who excels at the best for your own personal health?

Client: I believe I have interference from something that gets in the way.

TZ: Well then, let's tell the interference to back off for now.

(Brief pause.)

Client: Okay.

TZ: Now, I do not want some spirit person who thinks they can be a guide to show up for you. Someone who just thinks they could be a guide. I want the absolute most evolved being to be my guide. So, let's ask for a divine and sacred guide who specializes specifically in your health.

Client: I have a very tall, slim female energy who is in white.

TZ: I want you to ask some questions to help build your confidence. So, ask your guide this question: *How is it that you are a specialist for my health?*

Client: She says she is me, but I do not believe it.

TZ: Tell this guide that you do not believe it and see what she says about that.

Client: She says that is why you are going through so many health problems.

TZ: Do you feel that you deserve to be healthier?

Client: I think some part of me feels I do not deserve it.

TZ: Right now, form a very clear question about deserving and ask this guide about it. Ask her to give you more information.

Client: The guide says I haven't experienced all the things that I have done to others. I have not been able to completely understand what others have felt or experienced before. She says I chose to experience all these things in life to understand their experiences.

TZ: Ask the guide if there is also an element that you feel you should be punished.

Client: She says I am not done. There is more for you to experience.

But I say that I am tired, and I am done! I have experienced enough.

TZ: Tell her exactly that about being tired and being done. See what she says then.

Client: She says I have to change myself and stop procrastinating and my addiction to food and to drama. If I can stop those things, then I am ready. That is my fight.

TZ: Ask her if your subconscious believes you have been punished enough.

Client: My guide is saying yes that I am not punished enough.

TZ: Ask your guide this: *What is the exact moment that is causing the need for me to still feel that I need to be punished? What is the exact moment causing that?*

Client: When I abandoned my people. It was many, many lives ago. I was holding a very high position and I abandoned my people.

TZ: Simply ask your guide if you received that information correctly. She will say yes or no.

Client: Yes, correct. My guide is saying I did not fulfill my responsibility. I did this in three different lives. It is punishment.

TZ: Ask your guide this. Where is the punishment coming from? Sort that out with her (guide).

Client: It is coming from the people that I abandoned. I took a shortcut and did not fulfill my role. I left in three past lives.

TZ: Ask her if it is okay to show you the most important past life that is causing your current struggles now.

Client: I was a high priestess and was tired, and I chose to die very young. I was in a mausoleum. I was surrounded by lots of people, and they were pleading for me to stay but I left them anyway.

TZ: Now check to see if this feels right to you. Would you and this guide call in a guide who specializes in healing this moment and completely and permanently heal this moment. Make this very clear request and restate your command to this:

Completely and permanently heal that past life moment in time to heal you but also every single person who was affected by that decision you made in that past life moment. Make sure you ask for a complete and permanent healing for them at that exact same moment. Take your time.

Client: Quan Yin has come. I perceived the violet light spreading from my body to all those people and then it rippled out to generations and generations.

TZ: Oh beautiful! Now, if it feels right to you, ask the people of that moment to realize that the healing is for them. Direct those people to feel the ripples of healing through them and through all generations. Now, call out on the behalf of those people surrounding you for specialty healing guides to come for every single person involved in that past life. Direct them to completely and permanently heal and release every single person involved in that moment.

Client: All those people have healed at one time in different ways. Some healing is for one moment and some healed for years. Some were short and some deep and long. People come to mind in this life who were in that past life.

TZ: Check in with your own awareness and see whatever you notice.

Client: I notice more acceptance. I am little by little accepting more and more. I am accepting.

TZ: Can you accept that a great healing happened for you and for the others?

Client: I accept that I can make things right now and that they are all going to be fine.

TZ: You had originally stated that you abandoned people in three lives. I want you to do all these same steps on your own for the other two lives. You know now what the steps are and can do this for yourself and the others. Your block is that you have convinced yourself in your mind that you need to be punished and there was no way out of it. Now, you have just shifted this into healing. You have shifted this from punishment to healing. The thing that is most important is that we do not need to know every single thing about the past life event. We do not need to suffer again to relive it. We simply need to know that there are causes, and you send the healing directly to each cause.

Client: Some things are just clicking for me now.

Here is another past life example that this client allowed me to share with you.

Client: I just cannot believe that people do not get it. They are not noticing what I notice. They don't even live the way I live. They are struggling so much. They do not realize they have guides. I feel like I have to carry them on my back to help them out. I am responsible for so many people. It's like they just don't get it. What the hell? (Tearful and angry.)

TZ: Other people are not living at the level of awareness that you are living at. You are not allowing everyone around you to have their own choices in their lives. You are not supposed to carry them around with you. It is best to observe people around you. Begin to see them right now as souls that are living at their own level of awareness. You cannot drag them along with you. They cannot understand life at the spiritual level.

Client: It seems like a huge lesson. This grief reminds me of one of my past lives where I was speaking out against the government and my daughter was killed because of me doing that. My guides have shown other past lives to me where I took a strong stand against things. I feel like I have had this throughout my current life now.

TZ: Let's form a clear question to your guides to get a better understanding of this struggle. Let's form a clear, precise question to ask your guides. For example, ask your sacred guides: What would be the best way for you to learn your lessons that began in your past lives to help you now? Form the question in your words, however.

Client: I asked them this question: *What would be the best way to learn to follow my ethical and moral compass in this life?* The guides said it can be easy but not necessarily painless. They are saying to follow my own compass and what is right for me. They said it can feel isolating, but it can be inspiring to others and to myself. But this is causing so much pain for me.

TZ: So, rather than carry responsibility of these people on your back, you are to live your own life and state what is right for you and that in itself will be inspiring to many others. Ask your guides right now: What needs to be healed and released from your past lives?

Client: In my Turkish life I made a vow that I sacrifice myself to do for others. (Tearful again.)

TZ: When we have so much emotion about something, it is a powerful signal that we need to clean, clear, heal, and release something.

To accomplish a past life healing and release, you must realize that the experience will always feel completely like imagination or a great period piece movie. It will seem more like imagination than any of the other healing steps you have done throughout this book. Merely direct yourself to do each step no matter how strange or unreal it seems to be. At the same time, however, allow each step to progress as it wants to. Do not try to change it in any way. Remember, it is like a movie that you are choosing to view.

Steps to Heal and Release Past Life Trauma

1. Command to your divine and sacred medical intuitive guides: *Show me or tell me now the exact point of origin causing (name the issue) in my life.*

2. A situation unfolds like a movie in your mind. The sur-
    roundings and your clothing appear to be from a different
    time. Observe the details of the scenes with fascination but
    no judgment.

3. Send your current self back in time into that scene with
    your past-life self. Make sure that your past-life self knows
    you are there for him/her now.

4. You and your past-life self call in divine and sacred medical
    intuitive specialists and both of you command together:
    *Completely and permanently remove all forms of negativity from
    this past life moment, from our bodies, from our energy fields,
    from our spirit, and remove all forms of negativity from all
    timelines moving forward and backward. Remove it all from both
    of us now!*

5. In your mind's eye, watch everything that happens because
    of your commands.

6. When all the negativity is removed, then both of you
    command: *Great sacred healers come to us now and fill every
    single space and place and throughout all timelines, with
    unconditional love and the Light of the Eternal Divine.*

7. Directly ask your past-life self if he/she needs any other
    healing. If you receive a "Yes, there is something else," then
    ask what it is and repeat the process for the other issue.

8. If you receive a "No, the healing is complete," then com-
    pletely leave your past life self in that life. Release that
    moment and draw yourself back to your current body. (Do
    not ever bring your past-life self back to your current life.
    The past-life self cannot possibly be as advanced as you
    currently are now, and you do not want bring an unevolved
    part of you back to this current life. I hope that makes sense
    to you.)

Past Life Patterns Keep Repeating

Patterns that began in a past life keep repeating until the emotions within it are healed and released. Here is the next example from an actual session.

Client: I have done a lot of work about speaking to groups. I was recently asked by someone to explain something to the group. I said to myself, "Oh finally, I get to speak in front of a group!" but when I began, my voice started shaking and I began to nearly cry. I thought I could do it, but suddenly the group seemed too large to me. Is this about my throat chakra?

TZ: I want you to ask your guides a question, but you must put it in a very simple direct question about this struggle. Each word in a question to our specialty guides must be direct and clear.

Client: (To her guides) What caused me to be unable to speak in front of this group? (Brief pause as she received the pop of information.) The first thing that popped was a past life. I was shown speaking in front of groups and it didn't end well for me. (Emotional pause.) I was taken off the stage screaming, and they cut my tongue off. I still keep feeling like I am getting it wrong. I am getting it wrong.

TZ: Where did this happen?

Client: It seems one hundred years ago in a market square. If that is what happened, how do I tell my body and emotions how to heal this. I am at a stage now that I am afraid of saying things wrong. I simply freeze.

TZ: Let's do the steps to heal a past-life trauma. I want you to send your current self back to that moment and just look around.

Client: I am back at 1928. She is on the stage and she has a message for the people. This is weird. I see a fox. It is really fuzzy. My past life self is speaking, and the people are expressing, "Yeah, rah!"

TZ: I want you to call out to your divine and sacred specialists who excel in healing past lives and see who comes forward.

Client: There are three guides. It is like a dream and the fox is still there. Tell me now exactly why the fox is there. Is the fox a power animal for me . . . I get a yes.

TZ: Ask your guides to bring forward a healing while you are standing on the stage with your past-life self.

Client: This is so weird. The fox is now flying around in the air with a wand, dressed in pink pajamas. (Laughing.)

TZ: (Laughing too.) Power animals do things like that. Please accept that. It brings a delight to that moment in your past. Now help your past-life self. I want you both to take all the horrible trauma out of your past-life self and out of your current self. Get it all out and give it back to the government, give it back to the people standing there, and give it back to everyone. Get it out of both of you and give all the horrible trauma back to whoever caused it. Make sure you get it all and help your past-life self as well.

Client: I blasted it all out with a firehose. I got it all.

TZ: Ask that a cleansing filter be created for you and your past-life self. Do not create it yourself. It will be more powerful if the specialty guides create it for us.

Now, command that everything that was taken from you comes back to you now through the filter, all cleaned off. Purposefully put the purest form of you back into your past life self and your current self. You lost your confidence and your speech, and your tongue. Bring back anything else you can think of that you lost. It can be words or anything that you feel you lost in that moment.

Client: I also brought back my self-love, self-worth, filled myself with light, love, passion, and honorability.

TZ: What about taking back the sound of your voice? And ask your guides if you got everything back that you lost in that trauma.

Client: They said I did not get everything. I need to take back respect, independence . . . (long pause).

TZ: Now here is the next step. Feel your strength and look every single person in the eyes, and especially the person who actually cut out your tongue. Look all of them directly in the eye, feeling all of your power until the wrongdoers do something differently.

Client: They are shrinking and turning into mice and running away. Okay, it is now just me and my past-life self on the stage.

TZ: Ask your past-life self if you can leave her there now, very healthy, and you leave and bring your healed self back to your current time.

Client: The back of my head and neck feels different sensations of lightness.

You may find a common thread that repeats throughout multiple lives. For example, I often hear from an individual in spirit who committed suicide that they have committed suicide in many of their past lives. They will tell me to inform their loved one that they deeply regret their actions but feel as if they had no other options. Many living clients will tell me that they keep repeating the same mistakes as they made in past lives such as remaining in poverty, marrying the same abusive person, or getting caught up in jealousy, just to name a few. It seems that a pattern becomes more ingrained as subsequent lives are lived. It is like a rut was created a long, long time ago and each time the person comes into the next life, the rut is dug deeper. So, when requesting the exact inception point of your pattern, you will frequently be taken back to a very specific past life where the original pattern began.

While I no longer do this, I facilitated past life regressions for many years. I am a certified clinical hypnotherapist and specialized in past-life regressions. One client came to me because he was terrified to speak in front of groups of people. He could not understand why he could not do this because in all other areas of his life he was quite confident and successful. He said he absolutely could not get through this terror, and he needed this skill to move forward in his business and in his life. Immediately, in his regression, this confident businessman found himself in a shocking past-life situation. He was in the physical body of a woman. That in itself surprised him, but the woman that he was then was captured by Native Americans. He witnessed himself enduring multiple traumas of being raped, then severely beaten and "paraded around like a prize on display" in front of a large group of people watching him.

He carried the emotions of that traumatic past life forward into other lives and now in his current life. Horrific pain, humiliation, and extreme fear was entrenched into his essence. Needing to speak in front of groups of people in his current life triggered this ancient memory of emotions. Healing and releasing moments of the past liberates you from old, old patterns in your current life. The past could have been last week or many lives ago.

Negative and weighty thoughts and emotions move from one past life to the next, and then the next, until it shows up in your current life. Then you repeat the patterns because the negative vibrations are so heavy and dense that the burden of them show up in our interactions, decisions, and the way we live our lives. Those negative emotions follow along with the essence of our soul into the next life because we are trying to learn and advance, but instead we often just get caught up in the old patterns because of their heavy burden.

Heal and Release Vows

Science has discovered that our focused thoughts can imprint onto objects and have the ability to move objects such as metal pinballs. "Intent" is another word for focused thought. I have attended workshops where the instructor simply said, "Now set your intent." At that time I had no idea what that meant, how to do it, or what implications intent even encompassed.

Vows are real. If our thoughts and our spoken words move pinballs in a research experiment, then our focused thoughts are able to create an intense energetic configuration, commonly known as a vow. A vow is a certain dedicated commitment or a binding promise. A vow has a distinct electrical vibration that attaches and intertwines throughout our eternal essence, our soul. That distinct frequency has the power to follow us from one life to another. Some examples of common vows people have made throughout history are vows of:

- poverty
- chastity
- silence
- servitude
- a certain religion
- battling for a certain belief
- battling or protecting a certain person
- dying for a cause
- marital commitment for eternity
- family commitment for eternity

Some of these vows could open up so many negative possibilities that I do not even know where to begin. For example, if you tend to develop spiritually faster than your current spouse, that person could actually interfere in your soul's contract or your evolutionary progress. That spouse may become a negative factor in your current life, and you may later divorce that individual. The vow had already been invoked so it will seem that the two of you continue in a negative manner throughout your current life. At death, the divorced spouse to whom you made an eternal vow could then become a spirit attachment to you. That person could remain attached as if going along for the ride and not develop spiritually themselves.

You, on the other hand, would be unable to achieve the higher level of conscious awareness that you had hope for because your attachment weighs on you and interferes with your development. Now, this is simply a thought-provoking example for you and does not necessarily resemble a traditional marriage vow of "till death do us part." This traditional marriage vow has an end time, which is at the time of death.

Vows create powerful energetic cords, linking future lives to our past lives. The energy of a vow or a curse tends to build throughout lives rather than dwindle because more people talk about it and believe it as time goes on. If our words create a pledge that potentially lasts forever, then our words can also be a powerful tool capable of revoking that same vow. Before we revoke a vow, we must know, as clearly as possible, the exact words that were declared in the original vow. You will know when you perceive the vow correctly because you will have a powerful sense that it is correct. One must then feel a powerful commitment when they revoke a vow. The revocation needs to vibrate with as much emotional certainty and empowerment that is equal to the original vow. Knowing and believing that we can revoke a command with a command will free us from the chains that may have bound us for centuries.

Healing Steps to Revoke Vows

1. Ask for the exact inception point when the vow was made and took effect.

2. Ask for clarity regarding important keywords used in the vow.

3. Each time you state the following command, also imagine the physical formation of the vow, such as an energetic cord, completely disintegrate and float upward. Imagine the sensation of freedom and liberation each time you command the following:

   I now completely and permanently revoke and release anything and everything on all levels relating all negative vows. I am now completely and permanently healed and free from any negativity related to that moment.

4. Repeat this revocation on a daily basis until there is a deep sense of release.

5. Notice even the subtle shifts or changes in your life.

Heal and Release Curses

Curses are also real. I often hear that a curse will not work unless the person receiving the curse believes in curses. I would describe the power of a curse in a different way. The receiver of the curse does not necessarily need to be aware of it. That person, however, needs to be vibrating in a similar frequency to the frequency that the curse vibrates in. If the person is full of shame, guilt, self-hatred, or generally thinks that life is horrible, then the person's energetic frequency will correspond or even match the focus of the curse that is placed on them. This energetic match will subsequently link the energy of the curse with the individual's energy field.

A stunningly beautiful, well-dressed aristocratic woman sat down with me for a session. As I tapped into her field, I was shocked to see that her face was overlaid with a deformed, grotesque, blackened skull. Wormlike forms and insects came out of the skull's eyes and mouth. I told her that an ugly black skull covered her actual face, but I did not describe the bizarre details to her. Without hesitation, my client stated that she had been cursed ten years ago. I asked that she not tell me any more details until I received more intuitive information about her situation. I immediately saw an older woman yelling a curse with an alarming degree of hatred. My client said, "Yes, that is my ex-mother-in-law. She has put a curse on me."

I have noticed one interesting issue regarding curses, either coming from a past life or in the current life, the power, strength, and intensity of a curse tends to escalate rather than diminish over time. How could that be? Its potency increases because people tend to repeat all the stories about a curse. With each past life and with each generation, people renew the story and re-experience it.. Discussing the curse continues to feed energy to it. The harm that comes from the curse becomes even more real. In other words, more and more people speak of it and usually embellish the stories. As a result, the curse becomes more alive and more potent.

Many curses originate from the hysteria of being tortured. An example that I can think of began in the 1700s with one of my clients. In one of her past lives, this woman was a midwife and failed to save a woman who was giving birth. The woman and the newborn died during the birthing process. The woman was the wife of the nobleman who governed that area of the country. As the midwife was about to be burned at the stake for their deaths, the midwife screamed out, "Death to all of your babies!"

While some women delivered healthy babies, a few women had miscarriages or stillbirths. In fear, the people of the area focused much more on the deaths than on the living infants. This focus of thought energy gave life to the curse. The tales of those times continued to thrive, and an expectation of newborn deaths rose. That fear traveled from one generation to another, making the original curse from a horrific, torturous moment in a midwife's life into a reality.

Healing Technique #1 for Curses

- The steps apply if the client was the perpetrator or the victim.

- Ask your spirit guide specialists to give you the exact point of origin of your illness or struggle. In this case, you will perceive the past-life situation when a curse was formed and launched at you.

- Notice if it feels accurate to you.

- Important: Go back in time just before the cursing event happened. Notice the moment before the trauma began. It may feel as if you are standing at a certain place before the curse was created. (You are going to begin the healing before the curse was created.)

- Call out to the most divine, compassionate healing guides. Strongly command: *Completely and permanently heal and release all negativity toward me in that moment before it takes place. Only love and kindness now prevails from that moment onward.*

- Repeat working with your specialists and the command until you are aware of the sense of complete release from this burden.

Healing Technique #2 for Curses

Use the Raymon Grace Dowsing Steps, which can be used to clear and heal many different situations or illnesses. You do not need a pendulum. The power of focused thought is required. Say them in the order that is stated below and all in one sitting so the process is completed.

1. *Permanently scramble all negative thought forms due to cursing on all levels regarding me, (your full name).*

2. *Permanently neutralize all negative thought forms due to cursing on all levels regarding (your full name).*

3. *Completely transform all that has been scrambled and neutralized into Divine Love throughout all dimensions and all timelines for me, (your full name).*

Not all curses are sent to us from another individual. In fact, I think that we humans are actually capable of cursing ourselves more often than others cursing us. Once again, the words we use in our inner mind and the words we use aloud are critical to our well-being and the well-being of others. Our words shape our existence. With that in mind, take a moment to really assess how critical or judgmental you are of yourself. Do you mumble self-hatred comments to yourself or call yourself names?

People also repeat mindless statements such as "I am poor and I always will be," or "Nothing good ever happens to me and it never will." Can you sense the power in these statements and how they may be considered as self-inflicted curses?

Healing Technique for Self-Inflicted Curses

1. Watch out for the negative self-talk that you are doing

inside of your own mind. Notice the exact negative words that you are using against yourself.

2. Notice this is a form of self-cursing.

3. Form a command that revokes the negative self-cursing talk, such as: *I now completely and permanently revoke and reject all negative thoughts and all negative comments about myself. I now fill every thought and comment about myself with positive Love and Light of the Divine.*

Healing Command for Absolute Self-Love

After completing the healing just described above, this next command will create a foundation for you to continue loving yourself and see yourself as an eternal soul. This command feels like a meditation to me. Command this at bedtime and in the morning. Feel your entire essence responding to these beautiful words. Feel free to alter the command to use a word such as Source or Universe to abide by your personal spiritual beliefs.

Only God's compassionate Love and Light and the purest sacred Consciousness completely fill every cell in my body now.

Only God's compassionate Love and Light and the purest sacred Consciousness completely fill my mind now.

Only God's compassionate Love and Light and the purest sacred Consciousness completely fill my emotions now.

Only God's compassionate Love and Light and the purest sacred Consciousness completely fill my energy field now.

Only God's compassionate Love and Light and the purest sacred Consciousness completely fill my higher self now.

Only God's compassionate Love and Light and the purest sacred Consciousness completely fill my spirit now.

Only God's compassionate Love and Light and the purest sacred Consciousness completely fill my eternal soul now.

Summary of Action Steps to Heal and Release

1. Be willing to reread the examples of past life healings above.

2. Do you believe in past lives? What do you already know about your own history? You can tell from what you are focused on in this current life. What countries do you love? What periods of time are you fascinated with and watch movies or read books about that time period?

3. What patterns in your life keep repeating? Many patterns begin in past lives. You can often find the source in a past life.

4. Vows and curses are real, and the energy of them builds over time. They can be healed and released for good. If your thoughts can curse and vow, then your thoughts can heal you just as easily.

Chapter 22

Cause #7: Your Ancestors

"Genes do not create disease; instead, the environment signals the genes to create disease."

—Joe Dispenza,
*Becoming Supernatural: How Common People
are Doing the Uncommon*

Someone sent me a very interesting post on Facebook from a person by the name of Chris Swart. I think you will find it as thought provoking as I did. He called it:

"Ancestral Mathematics

- 2 Parents
- 4 Grandparents
- 8 Great-Grandparents
- 16 Second Great-Grandparents
- 32 Third Great-Grandparents
- 64 Fourth Great-Grandparents
- 128 Fifth Great-Grandparents
- 256 Sixth Great-Grandparents
- 512 Seventh Great-Grandparents
- 1,024 Eighth Great-Grandparents
- 2,048 Ninth Great-Grandparents

For you to be born today with twelve previous generations, you needed a total of 4,094 ancestors over the past four hundred years. Think for a moment—How many struggles? How many battles? How many difficulties? How much sadness? How much happiness? How many love stories? How many expressions of hope for the future? Did your ancestors have to undergo for you to exist in the present moment?"

I want to clearly state here that I have added ancestors as its own separate category of the cause of illness, challenges, or struggles. I mentioned ancestors in my other books, but I neglected to give them their own category of causing illness and challenges. The more I hear from people about their ancestors, the more I recognized the need to address this as another category of cause.

I frequently hear from people who think their ancestors were also most of the people in their past lives. That is not often the case. Our ancestry is not about past-life experiences. Your ancestry, as we refer to it today, is more about the physical, cellular, and genetic characteristics that you have chosen in your current life. Those people were not necessarily in your past lives. Most people assume your ancestors were also your family and friends in past lives, but often that is not the case. It is, in truth, generally not that simple.

The people in our ancestry lineage help to compose our physical body in this current life. Your ancestry certainly impacts your body and existence but may be completely different than who you have been in a multitude of past lives. Again, emotions cling to us throughout our past lives and carry into our current life. Generally, physical body characteristics come down through our ancestors. This is not the same as your past lives. This is your current family history for the current physical body you are inhabiting in for now. Some of the ancestors could be with you in past lives but often they are not.

It is our thoughts and subsequent emotions coming from our

past lives into our current life situations that influence the genetics that we received from the ancestors. Emotions from our current life trigger our genetics as well. Thoughts and our emotions either turn on our genes or turn them off.

In his book, *The Biology of Belief*, scientist Dr. Bruce Lipton states, "Positive thoughts have a profound effect on behavior and genes . . . And negative thoughts have an equally powerful effect. When we recognize how these positive and negative beliefs control our biology, we can use this knowledge to create lives filled with health and happiness."

One more detail that may clarify a common false idea. Most people consider all their ancestors as positive guides for them, and they call out to and invite ancestors into their lives and decisions. Please do not do that. Just because they are dead does not mean they are positive or developed, and it does not mean that they have reached the status level of being guides or angels. When we leave our bodies, we pretty much take with us the level of awareness and thoughtfulness that we had achieved at that moment of death. Calling out to your ancestors for help does not define any status or development as a guide, let alone the status of being divine and sacred.

The Traumatic History of Your Ancestors

Our ancestors had much tougher lives than most of us. Some of our ancestors suffered such cruelty and hardships of which we can barely conceive in our modern times. Life was brutal and people's thoughts were raw and inflamed with emotions. Those volatile emotions travel down the ancestry lineage on a physical level of the genetics, but those emotions also follow down the lineage through the family stories.

Do you remember in the last chapter that I said the following?: "Those negative emotions follow along with the essence of our soul into the next life because we are trying to learn and advance, but instead we often just get caught up in the old patterns because of their heavy burden." Well, that is what I have noticed about past lives. We keep repeating patterns because the energies of the traumas linger with the soul.

Now we are talking about our ancestral lineage. In this situation, the energy of negative emotions follow along the genetic lines of the body that you and your sacred guides chose for you to live inside in this current life. Remember that science is finding that emotions either turn on genetic keys or turn them off.

Not only do genetics affect us, but the beliefs of the lineage do as well. Again, the power of thought. Many families have stories that happened in their ancestors' lives. These stories can be about suffering under prejudice, traveling across the world to save themselves, or thousands of other situations. Families tell their stories over and over again. Another example of a story is that, generations ago, someone put a curse on the family and that is why we always struggle in such and such way. Those stories become intense beliefs. Beliefs have emotions interwoven within the history or the beliefs. You would think that as each generation moves on to the next generation, the family stories of hardships, curses, and beliefs would subside, but in fact they build with each generation. What family beliefs hold you back or cause you illness or challenges? You can heal and release these negative stories for yourself and your entire ancestry.

This client shares her ancestor's struggles.

Client: I ruminate. I can get dark about things. I think it is how I was set up astrologically or with my ancestry.

TZ: There are steps to take and we have the ability to heal our ancestry and our past.

Client: Ooh, wow!

TZ: Oh my goodness, that sounds like you really like that idea. So, let's begin with you calling in a divine and sacred guide who specializes in healing and releasing struggles through the ancestry. I will be quiet and put that call out to the universe and see who responds to your call.

Client: Okay. It is a native American, and he is huge! Nearly up to the ceiling and powerful. I feel him in my heart. My grandfather collected a large book of correspondences. They were pioneers and seemed to have no problems writing letters about the terrible treatment they did to the native people. Real sadistic stuff. I feel so much grief about this.

TZ: Ask your huge guide what to do about this history in your ancestry. Go ahead and ask him.

Client: (Long pause) I see this guide beaming tidal waves of Light through time and through souls who needed that Light. Then the Light spread to the Earth plane. He was pulling an old, corroded, rusty chain away from my ankles, and he was doing it through time. I had been held like a prisoner. I want to keep up this ancestral work.

TZ: Now would you be willing to talk to your big guy (the specialist she is working with) and take care in forming the command? Ask him, *Show me or tell me the exact point of origin that my ancestors' struggles began.* Then just wait to see what you notice.

Client: I see the 1500s, and I see a blond, curly-haired man. He is a monster and slaughtering the poor people.

TZ: Ask your guide if you are accurate in what you just perceived?

Client: Yes. I have always been fascinated with this time frame. I hope that man was not me in the past?

TZ: Now, stop right there and notice how you keep getting information but then you do not continue to ask more short precise questions.

Client: Yes, you are right! I do not ask the next questions.

TZ: Then ask your guide right now if you were the man that you were just shown.

Client: No, I was not, but I was born into that line. Your progression has been that you have been on the aggressor's side and the receiver's side. It is a dynamic that you carry. You will let it go . . . You will let it go . . . You will let it go . . . I am shown that I am put on a stone bed, and I am being worked on by spirit. They are pulling stuff out of me. I am being healed. It was a whole ceremony. Four Native Americans with wooden staffs were pulling all this negative energy out and spinning like yarn around their staffs. It was coming out of me and the ages too. They sent it up into the Light and cleared me too. The guide who yells said, "You will not have that energy anymore! You will do your work!" I think he means that I am to use all my training to help others.

Steps to Heal and Release You from Your Ancestors' Struggles

1. Ask your divine and sacred guides to tell you or show you the exact point of origin causing your illness or challenge. You are in some manner informed that it is your ancestry.

2. Ask: *How many generations does* (name the illness or struggle) *go back to? You will see a number, or you will count back through a line of people to show you the number of generations.*

3. Command your guides to show you the exact moment that happened to the ancestor that caused your problems.

4. Command your guides: *Go back to that exact minute and completely and permanently remove all negativity and all darkness from all people involved and throughout all generations from that moment, and remove all negativity and all darkness from every person who has ever been affected by that original moment now.* Watch what they show you.

5. Command: *Fill every moment and every person with compassion, benevolence, empathy, and unconditional love now.*

Summary of Action Steps to Heal and Release

1. You are affected by your ancestry lineage and also your past lives.

2. The same people might be involved with you in both ancestor lineage and past lives, but most of the time they are not the same individuals.

3. Remember you are only limited by the limitations of your thoughts. You and your guides are entirely skilled and able to heal throughout any number of people and across many, many generations.

4. Time is not linear and you are not limited.

Chapter 23

Cause #8: The Non-physical Spirit Realm

"The spirit world and the physical world are
interfused. The distance between them is the width of an
eyelid—and no distance at all if the *strong eye* is open."

—Robert Moss, *Growing Big Dreams:*
Manifesting Your Heart's Desires Through Twelve
Secrets of the Imagination

Interdimensional Experiences are Natural

You are a spirit right now in this moment as you read this sentence.
The aliveness within your physical body is a spirit. You are that
spirit and, yes, you and other spirits are everywhere. Some spirits
have a physical body at the moment, and some do not have a
physical body at the moment. Yes, dead people are everywhere
just like alive people.

The first time I presented information about the non-physical
spirit realms, in the advanced day of my workshop, I could not
sleep the night before. That morning, trembling in front of a large
class, I said, "We will begin today with the negative, but we will
not end this day with the negative. We will end the day in Love,
Light, and Strength." I then began to teach about the spirit realms.
I taught about the strange, the weird, and the negative.

As I talked, the room became extraordinarily still. The students
seemed to be immersed in my words. No one moved or became
angry or ran out of the room as I expected. I continued on with my

information in a neutral, matter-of-fact manner. The energy shifted when I said, "Many of you in this workshop are energy workers or professional intuitives. I know that some of you have had similar experiences to those which I have already described. I can see that awareness in some of your eyes. My hope is that some of you will now share what you have perceived. If you do share, you will help validate the details that I am teaching." Five students raised their hands to speak. They shared their own experiences with the strange, the weird, and the negative. The class then became eager to discuss this topic, and everyone began to breathe again.

Never chase away a non-physical entity. If you chase them off, they have to go somewhere. Most of the time they will just run out of the room or the house and stand in the yard. Sometimes they will run to the neighbors, and then those people are affected by the particular energy of the spirit. I see on television that some of these so-called ghost buster experts consider everything in the unseen world as demons and try to get rid of the spirits with hostile attacks or hostile words. Those methods only chase non-physical entities away and usually that is only temporary.

Years and years ago I, too, used to go at them with "guns a-blazing," but not anymore. I work with them as I do with any other client in need. I approach them with respect and courtesy because they are real beings. I totally consider all non-physical entities as clients. My non-physical clients are exactly the same as my physical clients. I approach them knowing that they, too, are struggling in ways that we physical humans cannot even conceive of.

My friend was driving to my house and still had about a three-hour drive to go. She stopped at a gas station for a few minutes, then got back into her car and headed to my house. When she arrived, it was late, so we went on to bed. During the night, loud sounds in the basement beneath my bedroom kept waking me up. I finally sat up in bed and extended my energy field down the stairs. As I extended myself down the hall to the basement bedroom, the banging sounds intensified. I stopped my energy field at the doorway of the bedroom and saw flashes flinging back and forth, crashing and bouncing off the walls. A sense of knowing washed through me, giving me information about what this was. I instantly saw in my mind's eye a young man around twenty years old being shot and killed. His terror washed through me, showing me the information beneath the fear.

I telepathically told him my name and told him he was very safe now. I projected calming, loving energy toward him. He felt the difference between me and his attacker, so he stopped flinging back and forth and stood still but looking downward. I felt the shocking, frantic energy drain out of this young man. I told him I was calling in loving, safe spirit guides to assist him. I asked him if he realized that he was dead and had left his body. He said no, he did not know any of that. I firmly directed him to notice his guides and tell me how many had arrived to help him. He said he could see two, and they looked like angels to him. I telepathically told him to go with them and do exactly what they told him to do. I saw, yet again, another indescribable release and transformation from earthly struggles into a dimension of brightness and love. I then went immediately back to sleep.

There is still a bit more to this story. The next morning at breakfast I asked my friend if she was wakened in the night by all the clamor downstairs. She had not noticed. I told her the story, and as I described the events her eyes widened. She said she didn't think much about it but when she got back in the car at the gas station and was driving along, something kept flashing in the rearview mirror. The flicker kept dashing back and forth inside of her car. She dismissed it as exhaustion and hoped she got to my house safely.

Notice from this experience:

1. My perception of the traumatized spirit person was clearly validated by the experience of my friend. I was so happy that I described my experience in the night to her before she told me about the flashing in the back seat of her car.

2. This is a perfect example of how people do not recognize information coming from the non-physical realms.

3. A perfect example of how people dismiss their intuitive perceptions.

Do these things apply to you? Do you now recognize and allow subtle information of the interdimensional worlds to be a natural reality in your life? Do you realize that this is all quite real and coming to you as intuitive information?

Yes, it is probably so much easier to ignore spirit beings around you and keep yourself in an unaware place, believing that we living humans are the only living beings around. Life might be so much simpler and convenient. But that is an extremely limited awareness and can possibly lead to being interfered within our daily lives and in our physical health. It could lead to becoming a victim to forces that exist but are unseen to many.

Positive and Negative Spirit People are Everywhere

I ask that you, from this point forward, now consider a deceased person as someone who needs or wants something. That is all. Positive deceased people will want to give you a message that they are doing well because you are their loved one. They will come to you to give a message to other loved ones. As an intuitive, they will come to you for help or if they think they are in need of something. They will also come to you because they are confused and really have no idea why they are standing in your living room.

My front door rattled off and on for three days. That door has never rattled in over twenty years. I kept going to the door to see why it was rattling, but it was secure. One night about ten in the evening the door rattled once again. I turned from the television and looked toward the front door. A man was looking in at me. Now . . . under normal conditions I would have truly been afraid to see a man standing at my door in the dark of night but at that moment I could see though him and I saw the tree behind him. I was safe because he was not in the living. Think about that.

I telepathically told him he could come in if he came in God's Light. In he popped and stood in front of me with his head hanging down. I asked him if he was the one who has been rattling my door. He answered, "Yes." "Why have you been trying to get into my house?" He shook his head and whispered that he did not know. He answered all my other questions with, "I don't know." My guides informed me that he died in a home somewhere in the area and that he had dementia, so he honestly did not know why he was there or why he had been shaking my door. Understand that something drew him to me even in a state of dementia, and take note that he still was carrying the confusion of dementia even after leaving his body in death.

I called out to divine and sacred guides who specialize in transitioning people from the earth plane to the highest place for his transformation into Light and Love. A peaceful shimmering translucent entity gently dropped into my living room, took his hand, and they both lifted up through my ceiling and were gone.

This is a frequent experience for an intuitive who is open to being a transitional assistant for the deceased. It seems we must look different or stand out in some way. We must also feel completely safe for them as well. Some are confused, some are still feeling sedated from a surgery that did not go well, and many do not realize they have left their physical bodies.

Last night a spirit person was baking bread in my kitchen. The smell was great, and she felt so genuinely kind. I assisted her by calling in the specialists to escort her to the most excellent place for her evolution into the light. That was much better for her than my kitchen.

Another day I had an extremely confused and needy spirit person beginning to interfere with my own mental health. Each day I too felt slightly unorganized and occasionally struggling to find the right words. This is no different than what you find in your own daily life. Some people are negative, some positive, and some are confused. It is no different than what you might find at the grocery. It is truly a matter of being aware of your physical world and the non-physical world at the exact same time.

This very intuitive mentoring client shared two stories about his encounters with spirits in surprising places.

Since Rick was a kid, he has been preoccupied with Vietnam even though he was not old enough to serve in the Vietnam war. He asked for my help to understand an unusual experience he recently had while traveling through the San Francisco airport. He said suddenly, out of nowhere, he was overwhelmed with thoughts and emotions of grief over that particular war. As my client explained this unusual moment of dreary emotions, he made a gasping sound because he saw a soldier in spirit come forward right there in our mentoring session.

I directed Rick to ask the spirit soldier why he appeared to him just now. The soldier answered by saying he has been with Rick since he was ten years old. The soldier went on to say, "Don't be afraid of death. You just pop out like you are quickly changing clothes. See with your heart and not your eyes." Then my client noticed that a Vietnamese woman with a tiny child and also a teenage boy all were hiding behind the soldier.

I asked my client to do the steps to assist them to go to the Light. He immediately saw Buddha full of Light and the woman and child went into the Buddha Light. The teenage boy did not go with the woman and child because he was afraid. I directed Rick to have a conversation with the boy to reassure him. I told Rick to convince the boy that it was safe, and to tell the boy to release all his old suffering now. The boy lifted up and away.

Then suddenly in this same session, Rick saw a man hanging from a rope. I guided my client to talk to the man. He said he began following my client when he recently visited New Orleans. The man had hung himself in a building that is now a restaurant. Rick had just been in New Orleans. The deceased man projected an image of that restaurant and Rick saw this in his mind's eye. The man followed Rick home to the east coast of the United States. I suggested that Rick speak to this spirit man who had hung himself. I suggested to ask the spirit person if he knows he has left his body and is now deceased. The man said, "Yes, I know I am dead." When my client began to guide him in the first step to transition to the Light, the spirit man loudly yelled, "No!" and zipped away instantly. Rick watched him in his mind's eye as he traveled back to the restaurant in New Orleans.

I always tell all of my mentoring students, "You just cannot make this stuff up!"

***

Remember how I keep mentioning that thoughts and emotions are beneath nearly everything? People, alive or deceased, are not really trapped in this physical world or trapped in the non-physical world. Really, no one is trapped. What binds a spirit is their focused thoughts and heavy emotions. People in spirit become glued to the same things they were focused on in life. They could be focused on their old property, a certain person, the sensations of being drunk, their place of work, the location where they died. It is a profound focus of thought and emotions regarding something in the physical world that prohibits a dead person from releasing the physical life and keeps them from progressing and evolving into the spirit realms.

Some spirits are causing or creating illness or struggles and they are not doing this deliberately or maliciously. A struggling dead person who is too close to our physical body can negatively affect living humans. For example, I went out to my waiting room to get my next client who was a twenty-three-year-old college student with an A average. I looked around the room and did not immediately notice her. I finally realized it was my client, but she looked so different. Her face was more rounded, and her eyes had a mischievous look to them.

As we walked down the hall to my room I noticed a man in spirit following about three feet from her. He was in full black leather clothes, chains hanging from his belt and pockets. He had a bandana around his head, and I could see his long gray beard. There was no feel of aggression, anger, or belligerence about him. I actually loved his "biker look." But he was connected into my client's energy field. Susie immediately told me that she was missing a lot of classes and has been thinking about dropping out of college. I looked at the dead biker guy, and in my mind, told him this was his fault. He said, "I'm not doing anything but following her around."

I informed my intuitively aware client that she had an attached spirit person corded into her who was interfering with her life and causing her change of focus from honors in college to dropping out of school altogether. I told her that the biker man was not trying to harm her in any way. He was simply interested in her as a young, desirable female. I emphasized that he was doing her harm, altering her values and her life goals just by following her around. I taught my young college student how to remove and release this interfering deceased person and together we called in specialists to help this spirit release her and be escorted to the highest place for his transformation into Light and Love.

Chloe, another young female client walked down the hallway to my office. As we walked, I perceived a spirit person who was a young, pretty, blonde female. This spirit was only a couple of inches from my living client. The location of any spirit, in proximity to the living person, is important to notice. The closer they are the more interfering they have become. I immediately knew that the spirit woman was interfering with my living client because she was only inches away. Now I simply had two clients to assist.

My client sat down and blurted out that she was suffering from a sexually transmitted disease for over two months. She reported going to multiple doctors, they all agreed she had terrible vaginal symptoms, but no one could find anything wrong because all the tests came back negative. As I listened to my living client, I watched my deceased client. Neither one of them had a clue what was going on. When questioned, my deceased client told me she had sex with hundreds of men. She then sent images of her favorite bar that she hung out in until her illness caused her death. I informed my living client that she had a sexually promiscuous spirit person hovering a few inches from her. I taught my living client how to communicate telepathically back and forth with the deceased woman just like a normal interaction between two living people.

Together we called in divine and sacred guides who specialize in transitioning this deceased woman to cross over into the Light. It is important to notice that I did not do this for my living client. I guided her through the steps to call in divine helpers to remove the spirit person from her body and energy field and then to call out for divine and sacred healers to come to fill every single space and place where the spirit used to be with health, vitality and love. The next time I met with my living client she excitedly announced that within 24 hours all the symptoms of the sexually transmitted disease were completely gone. She did the steps herself to heal the spirit and to heal her own body. That is what I hope to do for you with this book. You are powerful and you are becoming more and more in charge of you, your energy field, and your life.

Here is an excerpt from a mentoring session where I am teaching the student how to discover interference from a deceased person and how to assist the deceased to release and transition into the Light.

Client: I want to work on connecting better with my guides. I am getting a little better to get some visuals of them. But when I reached out to them this week, I got migraines for twenty-four hours, then I was vomiting. Something comes in the way. I don't know if it is a blockage that I am creating, but something gets in the way every time.

TZ: Your guides will never make you sick!

Client: When I go to get into it (to do medical intuition), then it feels like there is a lot of stuff that gets in the way.

TZ: Do I have permission to check into your energy field?

Client: Yes, you always have permission.

TZ: Okay. Give me a moment . . . (I check into this person's energy to see what is happening.) You have an interference. You have a person in spirit who is a young male, thin, with a long neck. He is corded into the back of your head. Tell me what you notice as I say these things.

Client: Well, I have been feeling a throbbing in the back of my head for quite some time now. I was thinking that I was self-sabotaging. I am having so much trouble trying to get to a healing center and so much trouble with planes and taxis, and now I am having so many problems with my children. Then I would have thoughts. Is this me causing the problem or is it something else?

TZ: Exactly! Now my hope for today is that you make a leap into trusting yourself. Listen to what you just said. "Is that me or something else?" That thought leaping in from out of nowhere is an intuitive signal to you that it is something else. Let's ask this man some questions and see what pops into your head. When something pops into your head, that is the deceased man answering. Ask him, "Do you know that you are not alive anymore?"

Client: I get a "No" from him. He does not know he is dead.

TZ: I had to command that he show himself. Many times, a negative deceased person will try to hide, but if you command spirits, they must show themselves. Ask him to tell you his name.

Client: He says, "Jeff."

TZ: Ask him how long he has been with you.

Client: He says, "Three weeks."

TZ: Ask him if he realizes he is causing you a great deal of interference in your life.

Client: He says, "No, I do not realize that."

TZ: So, Jeff is not deliberately causing you problems?

Client: No, he is not doing it on purpose. Now, I feel a heaviness at the back of my head.

TZ: Jeff, why are you corded into Mary?

Client: I see a tube from my head to him and he is lighting up from it.

TZ: Let's both call in transitional specialists to assist Jeff.

Client: He says five angels have come to help him.

TZ: Let's both tell him that he needs to pay all his attention to these angels who have come to help. You tell him that he is to lift up and out of you and go with the angels. Mary, your job now is to call in your own healing specialists to assist you to push him out of your body and your energy field. Command that every single bit of him is completely and permanently removed from you.

(Long pause of silence.)

Client: It certainly feels completely different now. I noticed my head was moving as if the healers were checking me. They are removing things that look like worms.

TZ: Now, I have a strong guideline that when anything negative leaves our body and energy field, I want you to command your healers to fill every single space and place where the negative used to be with Light, Love, vitality, and health.

Client: Oh, my goodness, that feels so different now!

TZ: Please ask your guides exactly what allowed this man in spirit to be attracted to you in the first place.

Client: They say I have a hole in my aura.

TZ: Repeat this command: *Give me now the exact cause of the hole in my aura.*

Client: They say the cause is self-sabotage by drinking alcohol.

TZ: It is important for us to find out what caused the spirit person to cord into you in the first place. When there is a negative spirit person causing an interference, the living person suddenly has a dramatic increase in struggles in their life. The struggles increase for the living person because the negative deceased person is very uncomfortable with anything positive you are trying to accomplish.

Most deceased people are not aware they are causing an illness or a negative life change for the living. Keep on top of this for yourself and your own well-being. Remember . . . as you scan your energy field and your physical body look for any foreign objects, energy cords, deceased people, nonhuman beings or negative thought forms lingering close to you or even connected into your energy field or your physical body.

Not all deceased people are confused, kind, or gentle but are still the cause of your illness or struggles and not all negative beings are human. This is a giant universe and it would be an over simplification to think that humans are the only beings causing illness and struggles. Some dead people and some non-human entities are mean, agitated, aggressive, possessive, and trying to do harm to the living. Mean, ugly, aggressive, and possessive does not mean they are more powerful. In fact, they are actually completely needy and weak. I see them all as unexpected, nasty, ugly clients who are in need of guidance because they have lost their way.

But even the most negative must be cared for with unconditional love and they too need even more help to transition into the compassionate Light of Source. All things come from Source. Everything from Source holds a spark of light. Even the negative beings come from the Creative Source of the All. From the confused, unaware spirit person to the darkest of the dark, all have that same spark of Light and goodness. They have lost track of the Light, have forgotten, or feel they no longer deserve anything positive.

Negative entities can be the primary cause of your illnesses and struggles. Your ability to be open to spirit being the cause of your illness will allow you to be an excellent medical intuitive for yourself. Any negative entity, at any level of intrusion, must be seen first and foremost as a needy, lost soul. Negative spirit people attempt to take power from others because they have no power of their own. They try to interfere with the living because that is what they were doing in life on Earth. They are like the aggressive bullies at school. But just like the bullies of the world, they have been abused or hurt time and time again. They have no awareness of love. They have no awareness of their own empowerment, and they have no memory of love, so they try to diminish alive people along the way.

You, as your own medical intuitive, must be commanding and in charge of even the nasty ones. You are still the commander of negative beings of all types and kinds just like you are the commander of the confused and kind ones. The negative, the mean, and the despicable will do exactly as you command them to do. They will follow your command because they are disordered, jumbled, and powerless. Negative and ugly does not mean powerful. It is the Light of the holy and divine that holds power. I want you to take a moment and feel the truth of this . . .

Signals of Negative Interference

1. You might find yourself making statements to others or having feelings such as:
   - "I have not felt right or well since I was at (names a certain location)."
   - "I feel weird all the time."
   - "I do not feel like myself."
   - "I feel like someone is behind me watching everything."
   - "I am having hideous dreams at night."
   - "I have gone to every specialist in the area and no one can find the reason for my illness."
2. You might find yourself noticing any of the following:
   - Instantly healthy one day and radically ill the next.
   - Sudden dramatic changes in your choices and decisions.

- Changes in your personality, way of dressing, belligerent attitude, increased anger and irritability.

- Sudden use of substances such as alcohol or marijuana when you had no interest for years.

- A sudden heavy depression or sudden thoughts of harming yourself.

- You feel that your voice sounds different.

- Your sexual behaviors have greatly changed.

Negative spirits are not powerful. They are just mean and often ugly. You, as the medical intuitive, are in a powerful position to assist everyone and anything involved. This might be a brand-new thought to you, but please understand. You in your intense brightness are glaring and nearly blinding to the negative beings.

Steps to Remove and Transition a Negative Spirit Person

Here are the steps to take if you discover an intruder in your field. No matter how innocent they may be, they could still be the direct cause of your illness or life challenges.

1. You have just discovered a cord or a spirit person in your energy field or in your environment.

2. Do not chase the intrusive spirit person away. They will go away for a short time but then return.

3. Power up your toroidal field until you feel that your Light is blinding. Telepathically ask the spirit person questions to specifically find out certain information. Ask each question then pause, and take what pops into your mind. That will be the deceased person responding to you. Your questions need to purposefully determine the reasons that a spirit person is interfering with you in the first place.

4. Questions to determine what your vulnerabilities were to attract this spirit person. Ask each question then pause to receive the answer:

- How long have you been with me?
- Exactly where did you find me?
- What attracted you to me?
- What do you get from being with me?

5. Next questions are to assist the spirit person to begin to separate from you. Ask each question then pause to receive the answer:

    - Do you know that you are dead, and you do not have your physical body anymore?
    - Do you know that you are causing me harm?
    - I am calling in specialists to assist you. How many do you see?

6. Command: *Divine and sacred guides who specialize in this particular spirit, completely and permanently remove the spirit from me on all levels and all dimensions. Take everything of this person out of me and take them to the best place for their highest transformation into Light and Love Now!*

7. At the same time, you push the spirit out of you and experience the release. Watch in your mind's eye as the specialists remove and lift the being upward and out of you. It is not only beautiful to witness but exhilarating to be liberated from the burden of an intrusive being.

8. Remember—When anything is removed from us, we must always call in your divine and sacred healing guides and command: *Fill every single space and place where that negativity used to be with cellular heath, vitality and* (other power words that apply to you and your own body).

Remove a Deceased Wrongdoer—It is Not too Late for You to Heal

For many years now I have sat with victims of abuse and trauma.

Hundreds are convinced that there is nothing that can be done, healed, or even resolved because they happen to know the aggressor or wrongdoer has died. I want you to know now that there is a great deal you can finally do for you.

If you had a negative relationship, negative experiences, or a violent event with someone who is now dead, it is not too late for you to bring a profound healing into your body, your thoughts, and your emotions. It is not too late to completely and permanently heal you and at the same time heal the exact split-second moments of those events.

Just as I said hello to Carol, my new fifty-year-old female client, a scary face of a male in spirit rushed between us. I instantly powered up my toroidal field and in my mind I said, "Back off and wait your turn!" He backed off but came right back and stood so I could not see Carol. I fiercely commanded him again to back off. He did so and remained about four feet to the side. I told Carol about the spirit man and described his distinct features to her. She gasped and sobbed. I softly repeated, "I am here for you. Take some time to feel all this."

When she could speak Carol whispered, "You just exactly described the neighbor man who raped me from the time I was six to about twelve years old. No one ever knew, not even my family." And then she said something very important. "I am fifty years old now and I still think of him every day of my life. It feels like he still rapes me every day." I responded, "You are not imagining this. He is still raping you. That is why he is coming in so clearly. But I want you to also know that is why he is rushing at me and standing between us. You are not just remembering events in your past and you are not imagining this. He is real and his actions toward me are demonstrating how aggressive and how possessive he still is. He is trying to scare me away so he can continue to interfere in your life." Her fear immediately took over and she yelled out, "There is no way to stop him!" I responded, "Oh yes there is, and I am going to walk you through the steps to take right now."

Steps to Remove a Deceased Wrongdoer from Your Life:

1. You are no longer a victim or a weak link because you are highly aware now of being the most powerful link in the system of healing.

2. Fiercely command the negative spirit person to back off. (Do not, under any circumstances, chase the wrongdoer away. They will just return when you least expect it.)

3. Immediately take charge of your thoughts and power up your toroidal field with rainbows, electrified golden energy, then fill your field with diamondlike flashing sparkles, then finish with stepping into a massive violet flame of Light.

4. Sense the magnitude of your power as you look the aggressor directly in their eyes.

5. Command: *The most forceful masters of the divine and sacred who know exactly about this aggressor! Come now! Encase and bind this aggressor tightly in brilliant white Light now! Completely, permanently remove every fiber, every tendril, every particle of his/her energy out of me immediately. Take it to the best place to learn from what they did to me now!*

6. Repeat the command again and again if you perceive the negative person fighting against the specialists.

7. As you fiercely command this, you must also push all the negativity out of your body and your energy field.

8. Call in divine and sacred healing specialists to fill every single space and place where the negativity use to be with complete personal power, confidence, and (add goals that personally apply to you.)

9. Notice the difference within your body, your thoughts, your emotions, and your environment. This is real and you just accomplished a profound level of healing and freedom. It is yours to have.

Be the Healer for Nonhuman Beings

This might be a stretch for many readers, but other types of entities inhabit the Universe—more than we humans can even imagine. When creation happened, it was apparently extremely creative! Once again, way beyond what even we intuitives can imagine. Just when I think I have intuitively perceived it all, I come across another entity that I have never seen before. There is much more going on in life than physical and non-physical humans.

Scientists had no idea that single-cell organisms existed until the microscope was developed. When each scientist looked through their first microscope, the world expanded in shocking ways. In the same surprising manner, people who open up their natural intuitive abilities become acutely aware of the extensive and surprising realms of life that we all live in, breathe in, and walk through. The mass population of humanity, however, has no awareness that anything exists beyond what their physical eyes can see. The physical and the non-physical exist in real life and surprises are truly everywhere!

Non-human beings exist, but not all are threatening or harmful. Some non-human entities are ornery and mischievous but do not intend direct harm. Some beings are part of the natural world of Earth while others are a natural part of other dimensions, other planets, and other universes. We are not alone and never have been.

I stood with a group of people looking at a waterfall in Ireland. Some people were chattering about everyday topics and some were soaking up the beauty of the environment. With a giant smile on my face, I watched the "little people." They scampered from rock to rock and then they jumped into the rocks. One of the rocks smiled back at me. Then suddenly many of the rocks smiled at me. The rocks changed form, adjusting to the different individuals that were jumping into them. The little people within the rocks smiled and laughed as some of their friends ran on top of them. This was the first time I had ever experienced what must have been leprechauns.

Yes, beings that are not human exist because the universe is complex and so full of life and all life is not human like we are. This complex life is negative and positive just like humans on this earth are both negative and positive. There are beautiful and loving people, and there are beautiful and loving nonhumans. There are negative people and there are negative beings. There is much more going on in the non-physical realms than is ever going on in the physical world. Just because we do not readily see it does not mean it does not exist. I want to describe some of this world to you to bring you not only relief but also remove all fear you might have about it. Once again, you are powerful and you are in charge—yes, even with the nonhuman beings.

I was a newly trained Reiki practitioner working with one of my first clients. She seemed deeply relaxed, and I was feeling profound sensations of love waving through me. I was a vessel of love and my client was soaking in the healing energy. I moved my hands from this woman's upper chest to her abdomen and felt a rumbling. Energetically, her entire abdomen split open and a type of gremlin leaped out of the client's body and onto the floor. It momentarily paralyzed me as I watched it run around the room with an ear-piercing shriek.

My only tool in my toolbox at that time was the beam of white light. The light hit the being and it too broke up into tiny particles that slowly floated up and out through the ceiling. I had not moved a muscle as all this took place. I still had my hot hands on her abdomen. I pulled myself together and completed a full-body session. I whispered to her that she could sit up when it felt right.

Her eyes popped open with a startled look, and she said, "What just happened in my stomach!" I could not tell her what I just experienced. Always being honest, however, I told her that she released a large amount of negativity that had been building up. She said she knew something released from her body.

I want you to be a prepared medical intuitive, ready for anything, at any time and in any form. I want to spark an understanding within you that will help you realize that you are not a victim of the unseen world, and you are especially not a victim of nonhuman beings either. The positive, loving beings are real and are magnificent way beyond our visions and understanding of them. They are exceptional in their strength and abilities throughout the realms and also exceptionally beneficial for us mere humans. You are in charge of you and your team. This transcript from a mentoring session describes how this intuitive woman is still having fears about the unknown. It is vital that she learn to be in her power and to take charge of non-human spirits.

TZ: I have been noticing in our session today that you keep bringing up the grocery store that you go to and how uncomfortable you are there. Before we bring this session to a close, my guides are saying, "What about the grocery?" Would you be willing to check that out with me now?

Client: Oh, it is when I go to the grocery or anywhere, what if I do see something? It does not mean it is going to get me! And it does not mean that I have to do something about it. Right?

TZ: You certainly do not have to. But in my experience when I perceive something, even scary looking, it only means that it is showing itself because it needs help. What is the scariest thing that you might perceive?

Client: The greatest fear that I might have is there might be something in the grocery store that I know is putting attachments on people or wishing harm to people or things like that. Something very sinister.

TZ: Would you be willing to ask your guide to show you the exact point of origin that is causing this scenario in that grocery?

Client: It is funny that I just saw myself jumping out like a superhero with a cape on, trying to save the world. (Laughing.)

TZ: Then what happened?

Client: Then I get overwhelmed. Then I go, "Oh shit!"

TZ: Well, what really happened is that a superhero is always alone, so you become very alone in the grocery store. Talk to your divine and sacred specialty guides to command the one that is the best one to work with you regarding the grocery. Ask that guide to show you the exact point of origin causing your concerns about going into that grocery.

Client: (Long pause.) Yes, there is something there (in the grocery store). I keep seeing this big energy in the corner and it is a dictator trying to dictate what happens there. I cannot even describe what it is. Kind of a mix between a big weird dinosaur and something strange looking.

TZ: Now that you are aware of it, what would you like to do about it?

Client: I would like to try to transform it.

TZ: In my experience, when I am out and about and I become aware of an entity like this, it is because it needs our help.

Client: Ohh!

TZ: Oh, I love it when people go, "Ohh!" I love that.

Client: That completely changes how I see it! Completely changes it! When I go in there, I see it as something menacing that just wants to cause trouble. But when you say it is showing up like that because it is ready for help. That makes it a lot less scary and intimidating. In fact, I just saw it shrink in size.

TZ: That is because it did just literally shrink. Now how do you want to work with your guides to help this entity in the grocery? Is the guide you have been working with the right one to help this particular being to transform into love and light?

Client: No. In fact, three other guides came in. (Very long pause.) Three of them placed it into a cocoon of white spider web and then transformed it. There was another crew of guides going around cleaning up the residue it had left all over the store. It was as if it left dirt wherever it walked around. So they cleaned up every corner and every crevice.

TZ: The fact that three of the guides showed up tells us a measurement of how negative this being was. When there is a negative being, it is best to command that it be encapsulated in white light, and in this case it was white strings like a spider web. This tells me also that this being probably would resist the specialists. You will be able to tell a difference in that store when you go back into it.

Client: Ahh . . . Thank you! This has been great and very helpful.

I personally have perceived all kinds and types of nonhuman beings. Some are wonderfully positive but many are intrusive if not dealt with. They can eventually wreak havoc or be lethal to those who are unaware. I decided to share with you a summary of the nonhuman beings I have personally witnessed or interacted with.

The positive ones have been some groups of leprechauns. I have seen gentle fairies and earth spirits. I have captured some of them in photos too. I opened the curtains one morning and saw two massive feet in the field behind my house. Even I did not believe my eyes for a moment. I looked at the feet then looked upward following the legs all the way to the face of a giant with a big smile on its face. I quickly pulled myself together enough to ask him a question. All I could think of was, "Are you real?" I admit this was not an in-depth question for an experienced intuitive medium who specializes in healing and releasing nonhuman interferences from people but it was all I could come up with at the moment.

Telepathically the giant looked down at me and said, "I am a traveler. I move all around the cosmos and beyond to other universes." I came up with a slightly better question and said, "But why are you here behind my house?" "I am a guardian. I am guarding you." He stayed in the same position for three days, and on the fourth day I opened the curtains and he was gone. That was about twenty-five years ago and I never saw him again.

I have also witnessed aggressive giant trolls, large drooling fanged mouths, snakes with a man's head on it. Once there was a satyr in my basement who told me he was from Italy. He said one of my grandkids accidently called out to him, so he responded.

Needless to say, I helped him quickly get back home. Three times I have come across beings that look exactly like Gollum in the movie *Lord of the Rings*. I could go on and on to describe many types of monstrous, grotesque beings but there is something much more important to discuss.

Negative beings, just like negative dead people, can create unhealthy interferences for humans that result in challenges and illness in our lives. I want to provide you with a profound change in your concepts of the negative nonhuman beings in the same way I explained about the negative humans. It is essential to understand right now that negative nonhuman entities are not powerful. They are deeply needy. Many are wildly ugly, but ugly does not mean powerful. They can and will occasionally create an interference in your life and your health, but that is not power. They have a neediness, or they would not approach living people in the first place. Does that make sense to you?

From now on I want you to know deep within your heart that any type of being that attempts to interfere with you is actually needy. That neediness is the opposite of being powerful. I want you to see them now as powerless clients in need of relief and in need of your help. Notice and feel the truthfulness of this concept and it will dramatically alter your beliefs and fears of the unknown.

It is crucial that you keep the following truth in the forefront of your mind. Even the unusual, the weird, and the ugly came from the Greater Universal Source. The negative has forgotten, ignored, or become fearful of Source's Light. This Light is literally the spark of life energy and knowledge springing from Source. Having the negative and the positive in our human experience gives us options and constant choices to make in developing our personal level of advancement and expansion.

Just like people in the living, some nonhumans are shy, quiet, and some are in hiding while others are aggressive, sneaky, or loud. Any and all negative beings trying to interfere with you are simply in need of help. Accept this concept, and you are on your way as an advanced medical intuitive to keep yourself well. If you are ever aware of a negative nonhuman interference in your energy field, you immediately become the commander and especially their healer. You are now the catalyst for change.

You will think to yourself, "Oh, there it is. I have learned about this and I am prepared. I am capable of enjoying the positive and, at the same time, I am capable of facilitating healing steps when the negative is interfering. I am ready to help deceased humans and nonhumans with my powerful knowledge and confidence in my divine and sacred specialists who are ready for my commands.

The following steps are designed to envelop and remove and release the negative nonhuman interference:

Steps to Remove and Transition Negative Nonhuman Beings

1. You have just become aware of a negative nonhuman being in your energy field or your environment.

2. Electrify your energy field with sizzling, bright, blinding light *and* the emotion of love and compassion. No fear, only more mighty love.

3. Command: *I now revoke, reject, and repel all negative beings and all negative energy that is trying to interfere with me! Divine and sacred specialist, who knows exactly about this entity, take over every element of this extraction. Now completely encapsulate this entity, and all others I may not have noticed, with powerful White Light of Source. Completely and permanently remove everything about this being from my body, my energy field, and from all aspects of my life now! Take it to the best place for its transformation into Light and Love.*

4. Be an active participant by pushing this being out of your body and your life.

5. Now call in divine and sacred healing specialists. Command: *Fill every single space and place where this being used to be with cellular health and vibrancy. Fill me with joy, love, and Light of Source.*

6. Feel and observe the complete healing process that happens for you and the interfering entity.

Commands to Repel Negativity

1. *I give permission to the greatest, most powerful Divine Warriors, Protectors, Guardians, and Transitional Specialists to take any actions you deem necessary to stop all interferences and all sources of interferences toward me now, and do so across all times and all dimensions. Keep all negativity away from me and keep me away from it. So Be It!*

2. *I give permission to the greatest, most powerful Divine Warriors, Protectors, Guardians, and Transitional Specialists to take any actions you deem necessary to stop all attacks and all sources of attacks toward me, across all times and all dimensions. Before they attack, immediately transport them to the best place for their transformation into Light and Love. So Be It!*

3. *I request the divine and sacred Protector of the Light to collect and totally remove all foreign negative entities, all negative energies, all negative connections from my body, my energy field, my soul, my silver cord, and from all my surroundings now. Completely collect them tightly in brilliant Light, lift them out, and take them to the best place for their transformation into Light and Love. Fill and illuminate me with brilliant white Light. Plug and fill all of the holes and tunnels in me and all of my surroundings with brilliant White Light of Source.*

The most important and vital realization is knowing that you have not gone insane when you perceive nonhuman beings. You can now say, "Oh yes, Tina discussed this in this book, her workshops, and in her other books. I am not surprised or shocked. I know exactly what to do!"

Summary of Action Steps to Heal and Release the Non-Physical Realms

- It is natural to know and to participate with the non-physical spirit realms.

- You will receive validation of your abilities in wonderful and surprising ways.

- You and the Light of Source are powerful.

- Ugly nonhuman beings are not more powerful. They are, in fact, weak and needy.

- Telepathy is a natural everyday occurrence.

- The non-physical world includes the negative and the positive exactly like the physical world.

Chapter 24

The Eternal You

"Life should not be a journey to the grave with the intention of arriving safely in a pretty and well-preserved body, but rather to skid in broadside in a cloud of smoke, thoroughly used up, totally worn out, and loudly proclaiming, 'Wow! What a Ride!'"

—Hunter S. Thompson, *The Proud Highway:*
Saga of a Desperate Southern Gentleman

Discovering Your Life's Purpose

- Am I on the right path in my life?
- Am I on the wrong path in my life?
- What is the life path I am supposed to be on?

Hundreds and hundreds of people have asked me those three versions of the same question over the decades of my life. My guides gave me the answer to those questions. The answer is the same for me as it is for you. The answer to that question is really a question, and that question is:

What do you find yourself struggling with the most in this life?
Pause right now and take the pop!

When I ask that question, as the answer to their question, many people get frustrated, irritated or blurt out, "I don't know!" Well, when you can identify what is your greatest struggle in your current life, you will know what your path is about. For example, some might say they are jealous all the time and they cannot stop being jealous. Another might say they constantly compare themselves to others and always fall short and cannot stand it that everyone is better than they are. Another individual may declare that they battle with depression or some will yearn to dance on stage, or another might say that they ruin every relationship they get into.

What struggle or pattern consistently shows up in your life? That is the answer to your question, "What path am I supposed to be on?" If it is continual jealousy of others, then your path may be to feel in your heart that you are worthy. If you find yourself frequently comparing yourself to other people, then your path might be all about learning to be the individual you are meant to be. If one relationship after another falls apart you may be on a path to learning about unconditional love. Look for the repeating patterns in your life and you will find the reason you are attending "earth school" right now.

As I write this, I am aware that most people think their true path is about their career or is work-related in some way. They think that instead of working at the dentist office they should have been the dentist. Some might think, "Why am I driving a bus when I should be driving a sparkling red sports car?" Well, it could be that your path in life is to learn about the innocent heart of children and to keep them safe. It usually has nothing to do with a certain career. Our true path is really about:

1. Expanding, visualizing, and knowing your individual level of awareness is experiencing the cosmos as a living being.

2. Knowing the electrical power of your thoughts and emotions turns on and fine tunes your connections with the matrix of knowledge within the Universe.

3. Realizing you are no longer a weak link but you are now a powerful, equal link in the alive system of the Universe.

Which of these levels of awareness have you experienced

lately? Learning about emotions such as vengeance, guilt, anger, rage, isolation, losing friends, being a victim, or being a bully offers you choices. You have choices every split second of your life. Which path have you been choosing?

I have studied with Michael Newton, author of *Journey of the Soul* and *Destiny of the Soul*, in the Netherlands. He also accepted my case study, *I Know I am Going to Hell*, for his last book, *Memories of the Afterlife*. In *Destiny of the Soul*, he states:

> "In a superconscious state during deep hypnosis, my subjects tell me that in the spirit world no soul is looked down upon as having less value than any other soul. We are all in a process of transformation to something greater than our current state of enlightenment. Each of us is considered uniquely qualified to make some contribution toward the whole, no matter how hard we are struggling with our lessons. If this were not true, we would not have been created in the first place."

Are you excelling at being the most compassionate, unconditionally loving being to others as possible and giving yourself unconditional love at the same time?

You are Never a Finished Product—Alive or Deceased

Mentoring students so often tearfully declare that they want me to tell them how to totally heal themselves with medical intuition. They go on to announce that they know they can never do healings for others until they are completely healed themselves. My heart energy literally shifts, like it missed a beat, to hear someone proclaim that they cannot help others because they themselves are not perfect. I then respond back to them, "You will never be able to help anyone if you are waiting to be perfect. We are never going to be a finished product like something that comes off an assembly line!"

To be the healer, we must first learn we are a mere human learning with each other along the way. Mastery has nothing to do with controlling other people or situations. The true meaning of mastery is to live with one foot in the physical world and one foot in the non-physical world at the exact same time and to maintain that balance. To me, the true meaning of mastery is to be alert and deeply aware of your own thoughts, your own emotions, and your own actions. Living with a foot in each realm gives you a magnified, far-reaching view of life.

I have witnessed people leaving their body and witnessed spirit people crossing over into the Light. I have witnessed the most sincere, heartfelt healing as people release their old emotional burdens and their physical body at the exact same time, and yet a cure at the physical level did not happen. Over and over again I witnessed that healing does not have to mean the physical body was cured. True healing is more involved, more complicated, and more divine than we can ever imagine.

You are allowing your awareness to open and advance by noticing the very subtle throughout your day. As you grow more aware, you will begin to realize you live with one foot in the physical realms and, at the same time, one foot in the non-physical realms. That is the deepest truth about having balance in one's life. You live a physical and a spiritual life coexisting in an unwavering awareness that interweaves into one. You sure can continue to have fun and even more fun than before, but you cannot be superficial. You live a life of such rich attentiveness, and that richness does often include being aware of spirit people around you just as alive people are around you.

We are all ripe with potential possibilities. A foot in both worlds allows you to peer out from the inner self to see, feel, sense the spheres around you. We are to learn from absolutely everything that happens to us, around us, and within us. We are responsible for our entire eternal life. That applies to our past lives as well as our current life and our future possibilities. When we allow a healing to take place, for ourselves and for others, we actually springboard our energy field into a different frequency.

That vibrational exchange flows forward into the future, back into the past, and outward in all directions. The energetic change also flows throughout our relationships. This altered frequency signals the Universe that there has been a transformation in our awareness and understanding. Each transformation brings us closer to true compassion without criticism or judgment. Each transformation leads us toward different opportunities and probabilities for our future.

Within the depth of healing is an intricate, wakeful awareness of all things being alive and interrelated. You grow in mastery of your choices. No matter what you do, be the most mindful, highly evolved human you can be, and do whatever you do with excellence. No matter what happens in your life, the goal is to achieve a more amplified, expanded comprehension of the greater wisdom without judgment. We all have emotional scars from life. What is most important is the healing beneath the scars.

Witness and experience all people around you as struggling souls trying to learn. You are the spark of Source creating with the vibration of your thoughts. Every moment in your life is created by the focus of your thinking. You are creating right now. You can create or re-create part of your life, or all of it if you wish. How will you know that a healing has taken place? The most painful experiences in your life will feel calm, completely neutral, and will never again carry any emotional impact in your heart.

One day, at the beginning of a session, I said to my client, "So, where do you want to go today?"

She answered, "To the stars and beyond . . . I'm finally getting self-love."

The story of your life is in your hands . . .

The eternal story of your healing is in your hands as well . . .

You are writing your own story at this very moment . . .

Appendix

The Primary Commands from Throughout this Book

- Healing Command.

  My heart is a sacred space.

  My head is a sacred space.

  My body is a sacred space.

  My energy is a sacred space.

  My higher self is a sacred space.

  My soul is a sacred space.

- Tell me or show me now the exact point in my body that needs healing.

- Tell me or show me now the first step to take to release anger from my _____.

- What is the most perfect way to assist (person's name) now?

- Tell me or show me the steps to receive financial abundance in my life now.

- Tell me or show me now the exact point of origin that caused (name the illness/struggle) for me, (your full name).

- Tell me or show me now the exact point of origin that is causing me, (your full name), to have (name the illness/struggle/issue).

- Tell me or show me now: Is (name the supplement/prescription) excellent for my physical health? (Receive the answer.) Does it work positively for me? (Receive the answer.)

- I am so full of blinding light of Love that only the positive stands with me and everything else is repelled by me now.

- My most holy and sacred Warriors of the Light... Completely and permanently remove all negativity from my body, mind, and energy field now. Keep all negativity away from me and keep me away from all negativity. So be it!

- The most divine and sacred guardian, come to me now. Protect my physical body, my energy field, my spirit, and my soul at all levels and in all dimensions now.

Teach me to learn more through positive _____.

- specialty guides of wisdom
- physical, mental, and emotional health
- life experiences
- dream experiences
- powerful relationships with the Universe

Commands to Repel Negativity:

I give permission to the greatest, most powerful Divine Warriors, Protectors, Guardians, and Transitional Specialists to take any actions you deem necessary to stop all interferences and all sources of interferences toward me now, and do so across all times and all dimensions. Keep all negativity away from me and keep me away from it. So Be It . . .

I request the divine and sacred Protector of the Light to collect and totally remove all foreign negative entities, all negative energies, all negative connections from my body, my energy field, my soul, my silver cord, and from all my surroundings now. Completely collect them tightly in brilliant Light, lift them out, and take them to the best place for their transformation into Light and Love. Fill and illuminate me with brilliant white Light. Plug and fill all of the holes and tunnels in me and all of my surroundings with brilliant White Light of Source.

A Healing Command for Absolute Self-Love

Only God's compassionate Love and Light and the purest sacred Consciousness completely fill every cell in my body now.

Only God's compassionate Love and Light and the purest sacred Consciousness completely fill my emotions now.

Only God's compassionate Love and Light and the purest sacred Consciousness completely fill my energy field now.

Only God's compassionate Love and Light and the purest sacred Consciousness completely fill my higher self now.

Only God's compassionate Love and Light and the purest sacred Consciousness completely fill my spirit now.

Only God's compassionate Love and Light and the purest sacred Consciousness completely fill my eternal soul now.

Diagrams, Charts, and Lists from Throughout this Book

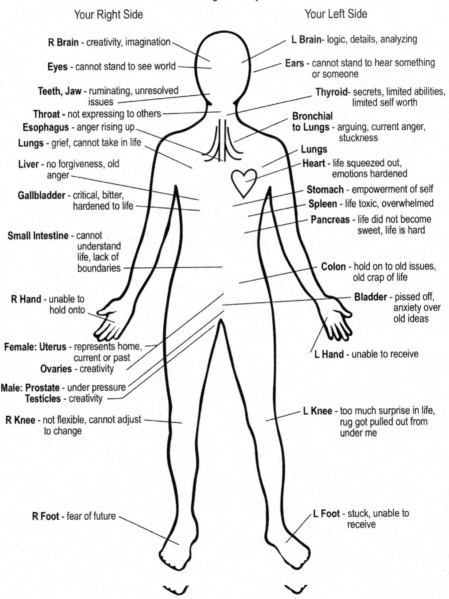

Diagram - Thoughts and Emotions
Affecting the Body

Your Right Side

Your Left Side

R Brain - creativity, imagination

L Brain - logic, details, analyzing

Eyes - cannot stand to see world

Ears - cannot stand to hear something or someone

Teeth, Jaw - ruminating, unresolved issues

Thyroid - secrets, limited abilities, limited self worth

Throat - not expressing to others

Bronchial to Lungs - arguing, current anger, stuckness

Esophagus - anger rising up

Lungs - grief, cannot take in life

Lungs

Liver - no forgiveness, old anger

Heart - life squeezed out, emotions hardened

Gallbladder - critical, bitter, hardened to life

Stomach - empowerment of self

Spleen - life toxic, overwhelmed

Pancreas - life did not become sweet, life is hard

Small Intestine - cannot understand life, lack of boundaries

Colon - hold on to old issues, old crap of life

R Hand - unable to hold onto

Bladder - pissed off, anxiety over old ideas

Female: Uterus - represents home, current or past

Ovaries - creativity

L Hand - unable to receive

Male: Prostate - under pressure

Testicles - creativity

R Knee - not flexible, cannot adjust to change

L Knee - too much surprise in life, rug got pulled out from under me

R Foot - fear of future

L Foot - stuck, unable to receive

Be Your Own Medical Intuitive
©2021 Tina M. Zion

Diagram - Thoughts and Emotions
Affecting the Body

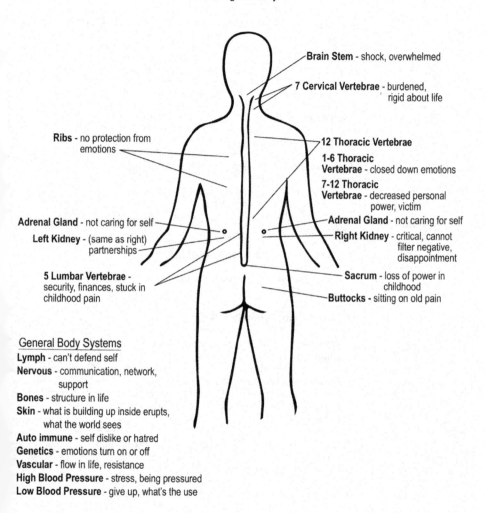

Brain Stem - shock, overwhelmed

7 Cervical Vertebrae - burdened, rigid about life

Ribs - no protection from emotions

12 Thoracic Vertebrae

1-6 Thoracic Vertebrae - closed down emotions

7-12 Thoracic Vertebrae - decreased personal power, victim

Adrenal Gland - not caring for self

Left Kidney - (same as right) partnerships

Adrenal Gland - not caring for self

Right Kidney - critical, cannot filter negative, disappointment

5 Lumbar Vertebrae - security, finances, stuck in childhood pain

Sacrum - loss of power in childhood

Buttocks - sitting on old pain

General Body Systems

Lymph - can't defend self
Nervous - communication, network, support
Bones - structure in life
Skin - what is building up inside erupts, what the world sees
Auto immune - self dislike or hatred
Genetics - emotions turn on or off
Vascular - flow in life, resistance
High Blood Pressure - stress, being pressured
Low Blood Pressure - give up, what's the use

Aura Colors and Meaning	
Red	Cellular health, energy, high temper, movement, extroversion
Light Red	Nervous, impulsive, passion, eroticism, sexuality, love
Dark Red	Willpower, masculinity, rage, courage, suffering, leadership
Pink	Femininity, longings, sensitivity, emotional, softness
Brown	Egotism, addiction, disease, earthiness, unloving
Orange	Active intelligence, confident, expressive, warmth, joy of life, sex
Orange-Red	Taking action, pride, vanity, idealism, desire
Orange-Yellow	Sharp intellect, quick wit, industrious
Yellow	Clear and active thinking, intellectual abilities
Dark Yellow	Timidity, thriftiness, restrictions, control needs
Gold	Devotion, higher inspiration, meditative state, authority, creativity
Forest Green	Abundance, harvest, deep level of healing
Green	Growth, change, nature, devotion, neutral state, healing, harmony
Light Green	Sympathy, direct, possible deceit or lying
Blue	Introversion, solitude, truth, devotion to spirit, wisdom, prayer, writing
Light Blue	Soft, reserved, religious, struggle to mature
Indigo	Healing ability, immersed in work, morality, spirituality, mediumship
Turquoise	Giving love to others in a healing capacity, expansion
Lavender	Mysticism, magic, overbearing, obsessions
Violet	Intuition, art, creativity, supernatural, imagination
Clear White	Eternal, forever, Godlike
Milky White	Spirituality, higher consciousness, physical pain
Silver	Love about the Great Mother
Black	Protection, shielding, detached from senses, negative interference
Gray	Low energy, depression, sadness, physical illness

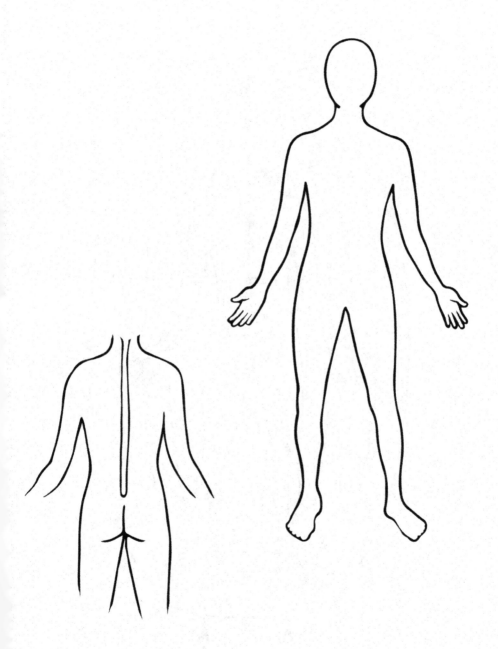

Be Your Own Medical Intuitive
©2021 Tina M. Zion

Hum

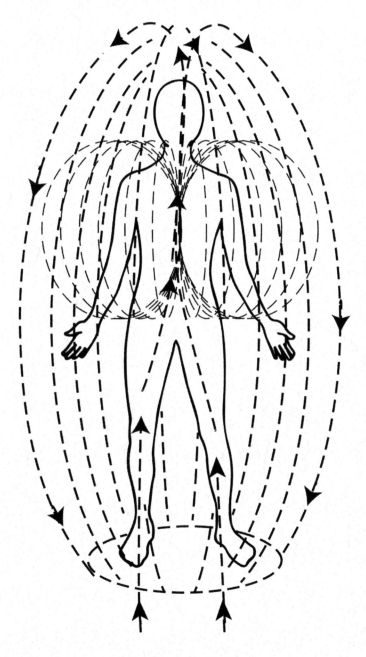

Be Your Own Medical Intuitive
©2021 Tina M. Zion

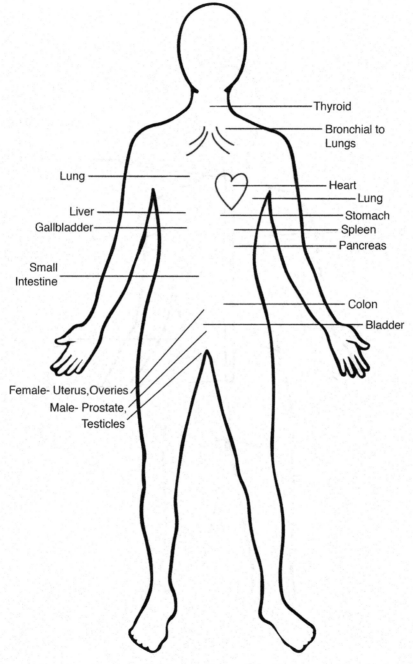

Be Your Own Medical Intuitive
©2021 Tina M. Zion

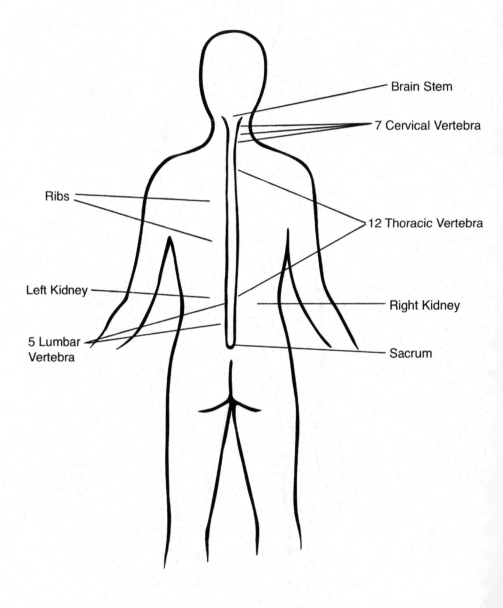

Brain Stem

7 Cervical Vertebra

Ribs

12 Thoracic Vertebra

Left Kidney

Right Kidney

5 Lumbar
Vertebra

Sacrum

Be Your Own Medical Intuitive
©2021 Tina M. Zion

Creating Scalar Waves
For Self Healing

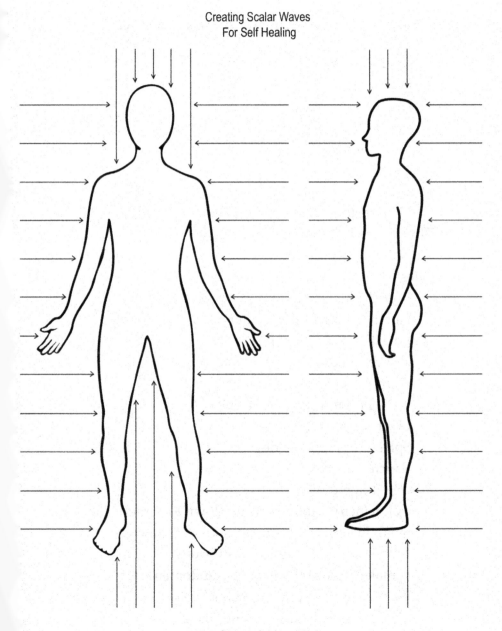

List of Body Sections and Organs to Guide Your Scans

- General View and First Impressions
- Aura/Energy Field
- Head
    Brain
    Face/Sinus
    Eyes
    Ears
    Jaw/Teeth
- Throat/Neck/Thyroid Gland
- Shoulders/Arms/Hands
- Chest
    Bronchial Tubes to Lungs
    Heart (slightly left of center)
    Breasts—male/female
- Upper Abdomen
    Stomach (center)
    Gallbladder (upper right side)
    Liver (upper right side)
    Spleen (upper left side)
    Pancreas (left side)
- Lower Abdomen
    Colon (across abdomen and down lower left side)
    Small Intestines (throughout lower abdomen)
    Female Ovaries (right and left sides)
    Female Uterus (Lower center abdomen)
    Bladder (lower center in pelvic area)
    Male Prostate (center behind bladder)

- Hips
- Legs
    Knees
    Ankles
    Feet
- Back
    Spine
    Kidneys (right and left side above waistline)
    Adrenal Glands (sits on top of each kidney)
    Buttocks
- General Body Systems:
    Blood Vessels
    Bones
    Lymph
    Muscles/tendons
    Nerves
    Skin

Your Action Steps to Heal

Simple Steps to Meditate and Listen

1. Sit upright, not stiff, but physically comfortable:
   - Do not cross arms or legs, lower shoulders, feet flat on the floor, allow teeth to part and rest the jaw, let your tongue rest on the roof of your mouth. Balance your head on top of your spine. Feel the alignment.
2. Close your eyes and feel them in their resting place.
3. Notice your thoughts with no judgment at all:
   - Welcome each thought and then release it. Do not fight against your thoughts or try to get rid of them. Feel the flow of your thoughts. Let your thoughts come in and then release them. Release each thought as it comes in. Pleasantly repeat this: Notice and release, notice and release, notice and release.
4. Notice your breath. Notice, without any criticism, each time your thoughts return to feeling your breath.
5. Breathe in the following manner:
   - Feel the breath move into your chest. Feel your breath flow all around your heart. Slowly breathe down into the depths of your abdomen. The muscles of your abdomen will move outward as you inhale, making room for your breath. Relax your abdomen as you exhale. If you wish, slowly count one and two as you inhale. Now exhale at a slightly longer count than you inhale. If you inhale at the count of two then exhale at the count of three, do not push your breath in any way. Only notice.

- Now notice that you inhale and pause for a split second and exhale and pause for a second. Do not make yourself pause. Only notice the pause in your natural rhythm. Inhale—pause—exhale—pause—inhale—pause. Now notice the stillness inside of each pause . . .

6. Now notice that you inhale and pause for a split second and exhale and pause for a second. Do not make yourself pause. Only notice the pause in your natural rhythm. Inhale—pause—exhale—pause—inhale—pause.   Now notice the stillness inside of each pause.

7. Your stillness is in the pause . . . Feel your Soul . . . It sounds different from your mind.

- Practice for 2–5 minutes only.
- Practice anywhere and everywhere.

Steps to Assess Your Medications and Supplements:

1. Have paper and pen to log all the details that you receive.

2. Sit in front of a large mirror to notice your own energy field.

3. Use specific, precise words as you question your guides.

4. Call out to your divine and sacred medical intuitive specialist who excels with medications. (This command will assure that you get the guide, on your team of guides, who is the best with medicines.)

5. Hold each supplement or prescription, one at a time.

6. Command the following: *Tell me or show me now . . . Is* (name the supplement/prescription) *excellent for my physical health?* (Receive the answer.) *Does it work positively for me?* (Receive the answer.)

7. Notice: What words popping into your mind instantly from your specialist.

- Feel your energy field as you command that question.

- Watch your field in the mirror.

8. Write down whatever you received and noticed about each medicine and supplement.

Steps to Create Scalar Waves within Your Physical Body:

1. Be playful. Take care to feel your natural empowerment first.

2. Decide the organ or area of your body where you want to direct the healing.

3. Notice the natural rhythm of your breathing . . . then focus on all the sensations of inhaling.

4. Look at the diagram. As you inhale, imagine that you are drawing energy into the center of your body from opposite directions. Imagine drawing in straight lines of energy from two opposite directions into the center of your body at the same time. Begin with inhaling:

   - Front to back and back to front.

   - Then down into your head and up through your feet.

   - Then coming in from your right side of your body and at the same time coming in from the left.

5. Think, imagine, and direct the straight lines of energy coming into the core of your body and into your head and legs.

6. Notice the serene, soothing energy collecting into a quiet pool throughout the center of your body.

7. Once you are filled with a still pool of energy, direct the still pool to go to the exact location that is ill or painful.

8. Be careful with the words of your command. Use only the most *positive words describing the results you want.* (Never include any words that describe the negative things happening to you. For example, do not use words such as pain, trauma, disease.)

9. Focus the positive command to the area of your body that needs the healing.

10. Continue your focus for ten minutes at a time.

Soul Retrieval Steps

1. Remember that intuitive information and intuitive energy work will always *feel* like your imagination, but it is real, and it is truly happening. It will become like a movie in your mind. Just let it unfold.

2. Stretch out and send the current 'you' back to wherever you find your younger self. Find the younger you just minutes before the incident happens.

3. Make sure the younger self knows you are there. How does the younger you know you are there now?

4. Take all the terrible energy out of both of you and give it back to the wrongdoer or to the traumatic moment. Notice what the energy looks like as you remove it from both of you.

5. Scan each other to make sure you got it all. Look everywhere to make sure nothing is left behind. Look around your heart and any injured areas. Get it all out.

6. Give absolutely all of the energy back to the wrongdoer or to the moment. **Important: It does not matter what the wrongdoer does with it. Just give it back.**

7. Call out to a divine and sacred guide who specializes in powerful cleansing filters. Command that a filter be created for you. Watch it appear and how beautiful it is.

8. Now, take back all that was taken from you and all that you gave away. Bring all of you through the filter so only the purest 'you' comes back to you. Place all of the purest 'you' back into you and your younger self. Make sure you get it all.

9. Take a moment to sense the complete wholeness of who you are. Feel your new empowerment.

10. Now with all your empowerment, stare the wrongdoer directly in the eyes until they change in some way. Hold your look until they change.

11. Tell your younger self to feel the complete healing of that moment.

12. Tell your younger self to permanently release that moment, come forward with you, mature, and then merge together with you.

13. Notice delightful changes over the next three to seven days as your younger self assimilates within you.

Guidelines to Raymon Grace's Three-Step Process to Heal and Release Trauma

- Do the three steps all in one sitting. You can do as many sittings as it takes until you feel or sense a difference in some way.

- Most people, including me, describe it as a sense of relief when the healings are finished.

- You do not need to know all the details of the past event. Direct it to all of the causes.

- You can use a pendulum for each step or not. If you do not use a pendulum, just stay with each step until you sense the action of each step subsiding on its own.

- The first step of the command is to scramble. Simply imagine the motion and action is like scrambling eggs. You are actually breaking up the density of the event.

- When you command to neutralize in the second step, you will feel all the emotions drain out of the past traumatic experience. You are actually removing all emotions from the event.

- The third step requires special attention. You must use the exact words that describe what you want the old traumatic times to be transformed into. A useful guideline is to use precise, exact, clear words that are the opposite of how you have been suffering. For example, if your traumatic past experience left you depressed and hopeless then you will want it transformed into joy and powerfully confident. If the trauma left you afraid of people then you might want it transformed into bravery with other people.

  - Read the steps first and rewrite them on an index card or paper and fill in the blanks with the precise words that clearly define what you want scrambled and neutralized and then the exact words describing the positive results you want.

  - Use the exact same words in the scramble step and the neutralize step.

  - Use the words that describe your goals in the transformation step.

Raymon Grace's Three-Step Healing Process

Call out to your most powerful divine and sacred specialty healing guides then command the following in these exact words:

Step 1: *Now completely and permanently scramble the exact point of origin when* (name the event) *happened to me,* (your name).

Step 2: *Now completely and permanently neutralize the exact point of origin when* (name the event) *happened to me,* (your name).

Step 3: *Now completely and permanently transform all that has been scrambled and neutralized into* (name the exact positive words that describe what you want), *now.*

Steps to Learn More About You and Your Relationships:

1. Imagine standing over at the outer edge of your life.
2. Observe like the most fascinated scientist.
3. Notice:
   - What does your life look like in general?
   - Who stands out as the most important, then second, then third?
   - Where are you located on the list of important people?
   - What was the exact moment that you lost track of you?
4. Decide if you want to change anything. You are in charge of every second of your life. It really is up to you.
5. Call out for a divine and sacred guide who specializes in helping you create your best life. Notice who arrives, and ask many questions such as:
   - What is important for me to realize first about my life?
   - Am I struggling to deserve a different life?
   - What is the first small step to take to live more in my own life?
6. If you decide to put 'you' back into your life, make the first step extremely small. It has to be a doable step that you can actually accomplish.
7. Work with this guide all day, every day. Communicate and communicate some more.

Two-Step Command to Learn from Your Patterns

Tell me or show me, (your full name), exactly what I am to learn now from this pattern of repeating again in my life. (Pause and take the pop of wisdom.)

Tell me or show me, (your full name), the exact steps to alter, heal, and release all negative patterns in my life now.

Steps to Remove and Heal Negative Cords

1. Call out for a divine and sacred guide who specializes in removing negative cords. Pause and allow yourself to notice or sense the guide who arrives.

2. Notice the direction the cord seems to be flowing. In other words, did you create it and send it to the other person, or did someone connect in with you?

3. Clearly command the following to the specialist if someone else corded into you:

   Completely and permanently remove every root, every particle of the negative cord out of my body, my mind, my spirit, and my soul now! Completely transform it into divine, unconditional love and send it back to the person who sent it, now!

4. Call out for your divine and sacred healing specialist and command:

   Completely and permanently fill every single space and place were that negativity used to be with vitality, cellular health, unconditional love.

5. You must actively participate with your specialists to allow the healing to happen and also to actively receive the goodness to come into you.

Three-Step Healing for Relationships

- Do the three steps all in one sitting. You can do as many sittings as it takes until you feel or sense a difference in some way. Most people, including me, describe it as a sense of relief when the healings are finished.

- You do not need to know all the details of the past event. Direct it to the causes.

- You can use a pendulum for each step, or not. If you do not use a pendulum just stay with each step until you sense the action of each step subsiding on its own.

- The first step of the command is to scramble. Simply imagine the motion and action is like scrambling eggs. You are actually breaking up the density of the event.

- When you command to neutralize in the second step, you will feel all the emotions drain out of the negative relationship. Neutralizing actually means removing all negative emotions from the relationship.

- The third step requires special attention. You must use the exact words that describe what you want the negative relationship to be transformed into. A useful guideline is to use precise, exact, clear words that are the opposite of how you have been suffering. For example, if this relationship is about fighting constantly, then you might want it transformed into unconditional love, understanding, peace. If the relationship leaves you fearing for your life, then you want it transformed into: *Stop now, permanent end of all connections with* (name the person.)

- Read the steps first and rewrite them on an index card or paper and fill in the blanks with the precise words that clearly define what you want scrambled and neutralized and then the exact words describing the positive results you want.

- Use the exact same words in the scramble step and the neutralize step.

- Use the words that describe your goals in the transformation step.

Invite in your most powerful divine and sacred healers, then command the following in these exact words:

Step 1: Now completely and permanently scramble the exact points of origin causing the current negative relationship with my state type of relationship (e.g. son, wife, friend), full name of person.

Step 2: Now completely and permanently neutralize the exact points of origin causing the current negative relationship with my state type of relationship (e.g. son, wife, friend), full name of person.

Step 3: Now completely and permanently transmute and transform all that has been scrambled and neutralized into (e.g.: relief, release, Divine Love, permanent peace, etc.)

Full Court of Atonement—Healing Yourself Regarding Relationships
(Developed by Amy Jo Ellis)

I, (your full name), apologize to myself for holding my heart hostage by demanding that things be different than how they turned out. I apologize to my heart for hurting myself daily, telling myself that I needed someone else to change instead of changing what I could control which is my own ability to choose to be whole, happy, and complete with things exactly as they are meant to be. If they were meant to be different . . . They would already be different. I ask to look back over my timeline and to call Full Courts of Atonement on all areas in my life where I took my happiness hostage and tried to ransom myself to force others to change. I ask for all of this energy to be corrected on the astral plane.

Full Court of Atonement—Healing Your Relationships
(Developed by Amy Jo Ellis)

I ask that I, (your full name), (full names of all others involved), all be placed into the Full Court of Atonement for the purpose of resolving and clearing all conflicts and transforming it into complete understanding, complete appreciation, and complete unconditional love in our relationships with each other on all dimensions and all timeframes. So Be It.

Healing Negative Patterns—Two-Step Command

Tell me or show me, (your full name), *exactly what I am to learn now from this pattern of* _____ *repeating again in my life.* (Pause and take the pop of wisdom.)
Show me, (your full name), *the exact steps to alter, heal, and release all negative patterns in my life now.*

Steps to Heal and Release Spirit People from Your Environment

1. Do not chase spirit people away. Help them. They need something.

2. If you do not see them with your eyes open or in your mind's eye, then directly ask your divine and sacred guides if there are deceased people in your environment? If you receive a "yes," then go to the next step.

3. Ask the spirit person questions and pause to receive the answers to pop into your mind, such as: *Who are you? Why are you here in* (my house, land, workspace, etc.)? Pause for the answers.

4. Then ask: *Do you realize you are dead? Do you realize staying here in this location is not the best place for you?* Pause for the answers.

5. Inform the dead person that you are calling in specialists to assist them into a new and special life.

6. Call in divine and sacred guides who specialize in transitioning the deceased and take them to the highest place for their transformation into Light and Love.

7. If the dead person resists, be firm and consistent. Keep telling them this is not the greatest life for them. There is nothing here for them anymore. Tell them to feel the love coming from the guides.

8. When anything is released, let it be filled and replaced with something powerfully positive. Call in the divine and

sacred healing specialists and command: *Fill every space and place where that spirit person used to be with Light, Compassion, and Love.*

Steps to Clear Negative Thought Forms from Your Environment

1. This is like giving your environment a good, long shower.
2. Call out to divine and sacred guides who specialize in removing and cleansing all types of negativity.
3. Command the following: *Now completely and permanently remove all accumulations of negativity on all levels and in all places associated with me,* (your full name).
4. Then command the following: *Now cleanse all spaces and places where the negative used to be with precious, pure, clean energy. Permanently place it within, throughout and around on all levels and in all dimensions.*

Steps to Clear Physical Toxins from Your Environment

Raymon Grace is very well known for using these steps to clean up and heal schools for children and for clearing toxins from water and land. Three-Step Healing Commands:

Invite in your most powerful, divine, and sacred healers, then command the following in these exact words:

Step 1: *Now completely and permanently scramble all the exact points of origin causing the toxic, contaminated* (name the land, water, or area, etc.) *at* (name the exact address or location.)

Step 2: *Now completely and permanently neutralize all the exact points of origin causing the toxic, contaminated* (name the land, water, or area, etc.) *at* (name the exact address or location.)

Step 3: *Now completely and permanently transform all that has been scrambled and neutralized into* (clean, wholesome, vitally alive, etc.) (name the land, water, or area, etc.) *at* (name the exact address or location.)

Healing Steps to Revoke Vows

1. Ask for the exact inception point when the vow was made and took effect.

2. Ask for clarity regarding important keywords used in the vow.

3. Each time you state the following command, also imagine the physical formation of the vow, such as an energetic cord, completely disintegrate and float upward. Imagine the sensation of freedom and liberation each time you command the following:

"I now completely and permanently revoke and release anything and everything on all levels relating all negative vows. I am now completely and permanently healed and free from any negativity related to that moment."

4. Repeat this revocation on a daily basis until there is a deep sense of release.

5. Notice even the subtle shifts or changes in your life.

Healing Technique #1 for Curses

- The steps apply if the client was the perpetrator or the victim.

- Ask your spirit guide specialists to give you the exact point of origin of your illness or struggle. In this case, you will perceive the past-life situation when a curse was formed and launched at you.

- Notice if it feels accurate to you.

- Important: Go back in time just before the cursing event happened. Notice the moment before the trauma began. It may feel as if you are standing at a certain place before the curse was created. (You are going to begin the healing before the curse was created.)

- Call out to the most divine, compassionate healing guides. Strongly command: *Completely and permanently heal and release all negativity toward me in that moment before it takes place. Only love and kindness now prevails from that moment onward.*

- Repeat working with your specialists and the command until you are aware of the sense of complete release from this burden.

Healing Technique #2 for Curses

Use the Raymon Grace Dowsing Steps, which can be used to clear and heal many different situations or illnesses. You do not need a pendulum. The power of focused thought is required. Say them in the order that is stated below and all in one sitting so the process is completed.

1. *Permanently scramble all negative thought forms due to cursing on all levels regarding me, (your full name).*

2. *Permanently neutralize all negative thought forms due to cursing on all levels regarding (your full name).*

3. *Completely transform all that has been scrambled and neutralized into Divine Love, throughout all dimensions, and all timelines for me, (your full name).*

Healing Technique for Self-Inflicted Curses

1. Watch out for the negative self-talk that you are doing inside of your own mind. Notice the exact negative words that you are using against yourself.

2. Notice this is a form of self-cursing.

3. Form a command that revokes the negative self-cursing talk, such as: *I now completely and permanently revoke and*

reject all negative thoughts and all negative comments about myself. I now fill every thought and comment about myself with positive Love and Light of the Divine.

Steps to Heal and Release You from Your Ancestors' Struggles

1. Ask your divine and sacred guides to tell you or show you the exact point of origin causing your illness or challenge. You are in some manner informed that it is your ancestry.

2. Ask: *How many generations does* (name the illness or struggle) *go back to?* You will see a number, or you will count back through a line of people to show you the number of generations.

3. Command your guides to show you the exact moment that happened to the ancestor that caused your problems.

4. Command your guides: *Go back to that exact minute and completely and permanently remove all negativity and all darkness from all people involved and throughout all generations from that moment and remove all negativity and all darkness from every person who has ever been affected by that original moment now.* Watch what they show you.

5. Command: *Fill every moment and every person with compassion, benevolence, empathy, and unconditional love now.*

Steps to Remove and Transition a Negative Spirit Person

1. You have just discovered a cord or a spirit person in your energy field or in your environment.

2. Do not chase the intrusive spirit person away. They will go away for a short time but then return.

3. Power up your toroidal field until you feel that your Light is blinding. Telepathically ask the spirit person questions to specifically find out certain information. Ask each question then pause, and take what pops into your mind. That will

be the deceased person responding to you. Your questions need to purposefully determine the reasons that a spirit person is interfering with you in the first place.

4. Questions to determine what your vulnerabilities were to attract this spirit person. Ask each question then pause to receive the answer:

    • How long have you been with me?

    • Exactly where did you find me?

    • What attracted you to me?

    • What do you get from being with me?

5. Next questions are to assist the spirit person to begin to separate from you. Ask each question then pause to receive the answer:

    • Do you know that you are dead, and you do not have your physical body anymore?

    • Do you know that you are causing me harm?

    • I am calling in specialists to assist you. How many do you see?

6. Command: *Divine and sacred guides who specialize in this particular spirit, completely and permanently remove the spirit from me on all levels and all dimensions. Take everything of this person out of me and take them to the best place for their highest transformation into Light and Love Now!*

7. At the same time, you push the spirit out of you and experience the release. Watch in your mind's eye as the specialists remove and lift the being upward and out of you. It is not only beautiful to witness but exhilarating to be liberated from the burden of an intrusive being.

8. Remember—When anything is removed from us, we must always call in your divine and sacred healing guides and command: *Fill every single space and place where that negativity used to be with cellular heath, vitality and* (other power words that apply to you and your own body).

Steps to Remove a Deceased Wrongdoer from Your Life

1. You are no longer a victim or a weak link because you are highly aware now of being the most powerful link in the system of healing.

2. Fiercely command the negative spirit person to back off. (Do not under any circumstances, chase the wrongdoer away. They will just return when you least expect it.)

3. Immediately take charge of your thoughts and power up your toroidal field with rainbows, electrified golden energy, then fill your field with diamondlike flashing sparkles, then finish with stepping into a massive violet flame of Light.

4. Sense the magnitude of your power as you look the aggressor directly in their eyes.

5. Command: *The most forceful masters of the divine and sacred who know exactly about this aggressor! Come now! Encase and bind this aggressor tightly in brilliant white Light now! Completely, permanently remove every fiber, every tendril, every particle of his/her energy out of me immediately. Take it to the best place to learn from what they did to me now!*

6. Repeat the command again and again if you perceive the negative person fighting against the specialists.

7. As you fiercely command this you must also push all the negativity out of your body and your energy field.

8. Call in divine and sacred healing specialists to fill every single space and place where the negativity use to be with complete personal power, confidence, and (add goals that personally apply to you.)

9. Notice the difference within your body, your thoughts, your emotions, and your environment. This is real and you just accomplished a profound level of healing and freedom. It is yours to have.

Healing Steps to Remove and Transition Negative Nonhuman Beings

1. You have just become aware of a negative nonhuman being in your energy field or your environment.

2. Electrify your energy field with sizzling, bright, blinding light *and* the emotion of love and compassion. No fear, only more mighty love.

3. Command: *I now revoke, reject, and repel all negative beings and all negative energy that is trying to interfere with me! Divine and sacred specialist, who knows exactly about this entity, take over every element of this extraction. Now completely encapsulate this entity and all others I may not have noticed, with powerful White Light of Source. Completely and permanently remove everything about this being from my body, my energy field, and from all aspects of my life now! Take it to the best place for its transformation into Light and Love.*

4. Be an active participant by pushing this being out of your body and your life.

5. Now call in divine and sacred healing specialists. Command: *Fill every single space and place where this being used to be with cellular health and vibrancy. Fill me with joy, love, and Light of Source.*

6. Feel and observe the complete healing process that happens for you and the interfering entity.

Suggested Reading and Resources List

The Biology of Belief by Dr. Bruce Lipton

Walking in Light: The Everyday Empowerment of a Shamanic Life by Sandra Ingerman

The Master Key: Qigong Secrets for Vitality, Love, and Wisdom by Robert Peng

The Empath's Survival Guide by Judith Orloff MD.

Journey of Souls by Michael Newton

Destiny of Souls by Michael Newton

Memories of the Afterlife edited by M. Newton (Tina is a contributing author)

The Fourth Phase of Water: Beyond Solid, Liquid, and Vapor by Gerald H. Pollack and Ethan Pollack

The Body Electric: Electromagnetism and The Foundation of Life by Robert Becker

Earth Grids by Hugh Newman

The Unquiet Dead by Edith Fiore

Beyond the Veil: Our Journey Home by Diane Goble

Sidewalk Oracles: Playing with Signs, Symbols and Synchronicity in Everyday Life by Robert Moss

The Dreamer's Book of the Dead: A Soul Traveler's Guide to Death, Dying and the Other Side

Imaginal Realm by Robert Moss

Dreamgates by Robert Moss

Healing the Chakra Energy System by John R. Cross

The Emotion Code by Dr. Bradley Nelson

Court of Atonement (e-book) by Amy Jo Ellis (AmyJoEllis.com)

The Body Keeps the Score by Bessel Van Der Kolk, MD

The Intention Experiment by Lynne McTaggert

Mind Mastery Meditations by Valerie Hunt Ed.D

The Afterlife of Billy Fingers by Annie Kagan

May Cause Miracles by Gabrielle Bernstein

Heal (movie), directed by Kelly Noonan Gores

Book of Changes: A Guide to Life's Turning Points by Brian Brown Walker

Molecules of Emotion by Candice Pert, PhD

E-Squared by Pam Grout

Learn to Assist People in the Death Process—End-of-Life Doula Class by Henry Fersko-Weiss (Inelda.org)

Discussion Points for Book Clubs and Reading Groups

1. This book defines medical intuition and states that intuition is a natural ability. How have you noticed intuition in your life and how have you possibly blocked your own abilities?

2. The author explains how most people do not recognize what intuition is when it happens in their lives. As you read the pathways and the real-life examples of intuitive information, can you more readily identify intuition happening in your life now? What examples can you share with the group? Can you understand the meaning for your personally?

3. The author describes how our thoughts and emotions are creating our lives. Is this a new idea to you and does it make sense?

4. Communicating with your own body and the universe and spiritual guides is emphasized in the book. Discuss what you have noticed, and has it been positive for you?

5. The author identifies eight causes of illness. Can you relate to any of these causes of illness that the author describes?

6. The author gives step by step guidelines to bring healing to oneself. Have you used any of these methods for yourself and have you noticed any positive changes in your life? Are you willing to share your experience with the group?

About the Author

Tina Zion is a fourth-generation intuitive medium, educator, and is considered an expert in medical intuition. She is an award-winning author, specializing in medical intuition and teaching it internationally. Tina teaches her course, Become a Medical Intuitive, in the United Kingdom, Europe, New Zealand, Australia, Canada, Mexico, and throughout the US.

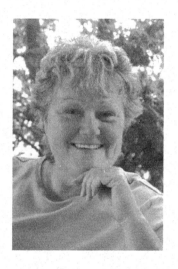

Tina has worked in the mental health field as a registered nurse with a national board specialty certification in mental health nursing from the American Nurses Credentialing Association. She is a Gestalt trained mental health counselor, graduating from the Indianapolis Gestalt Institute in 1997. She received her certification in clinical hypnotherapy from the American Council of Hypnotist Examiners and specialized in past life regressions. Tina was also certified through the Michael Newton Institute. She received her first Reiki attunement from Diane Stein and went on to receive the Master-Teacher degree. She taught Reiki for over ten years.

As an internationally known author, Tina's first two medical intuition books both won first place gold awards, and her four books are selling in over forty countries. She is the author of *Become a Medical Intuitive, Advanced Medical Intuition, The Reiki Teacher's Manual, Reiki and Your Intuition*, and is a contributing author in Michael Newton's book, *Memories of the Afterlife*.

Tina now focuses on teaching medical intuition all around the globe.

For more information, visit Tina's website at:
www.tinazion.com

Other Books in the Medical Intuitive Series

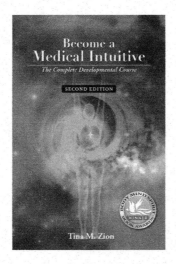

International instructor. and speaker, Tina M. Zion, created the second edition of her bestselling medical intuitive training manual. In this second edition, Zion places emphasis on:

- Developing inner sight for the deeper cause of illness.
- Feeling, sensing, and seeing the entire person on all levels.
- Accessing a person's eternal story for healing.
- Understanding the electromagnetic energy of thought and emotion.
- Assessing what vibrational colors of the aura are telling you.
- Doing distance assessments.
  And more.

This teaching manual is for lay people, medical practitioners, energy healers, professional intuitives and mediums, and anyone who wants to develop their intuitive abilities. This is an experiential process to learn and become a medical intuitive for others.

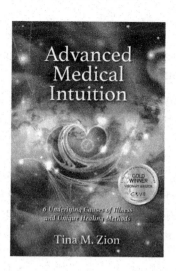

Finding the true cause of illness leads to healings that are far beyond the superficial level. Advanced Medical Intuition is power-packed with information. This book is the next step to take after reading Tina Zion's book, *Become a Medical Intuitive: The Complete Developmental Course*. It will enable you to use those refined intuitive skills to uncover the six causes of illness and the unique healing methods for each cause.

Finding the true cause of illness leads to healings that are far beyond the superficial level. This teaching manual offers these educational features for your success:

- Descriptions of the six causes of illness and the specific healing techniques for each category.
- Case studies transcribed from the author's recorded medical intuitive sessions.
- Case studies presented in narrative story-like form.
- Comments within the transcriptions explain each segment.
- Healing techniques are demonstrated in transcripts, narratives, and in numbered steps throughout the book.
- Step-by-step explanations describing purpose and healing goals.

- Key concepts are highlighted throughout.
- Different approaches to engage and empower your clients as the session progresses.
- A complete summary of the healing techniques for a quick guide to learn from. Take your medical intuitive abilities to the next level.

This advanced manual assists newly aware individuals as well as the professional already in private practice. Your successes and confidence will quickly develop as you take action with these intuitive skills and healing methods.

Other Books by Tina M. Zion

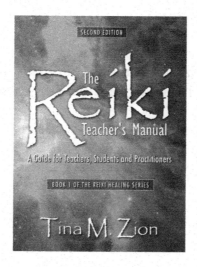

The Reiki Teacher's Manual (Second Edition) sets the standard for Reiki education.

This book is designed for students, practitioners, and teachers. This enhanced new edition will enrich the classes for current teachers and gives the new teacher confidence and pride when providing that very first class. Practitioners will have a greater understanding of how to apply Reiki and what is actually happening during a session. This manual provides:

- A quick reference to answer students' questions.
- Consecutive steps with time approximations.
- How to structure hands-on practice sessions.
- How to increase the power of your attunement.
- How to teach the attunement to others.
- Goals to achieve.
- Detailed descriptions and uses for the symbols.

- Fifteen handouts that are concise, informative, and can be copied from the book.

- A list of supplies.

As a practitioner, you will never be afraid or even worried about teaching a Reiki class or giving attunements. Your students will be grateful and confident for the rich content your classes give.

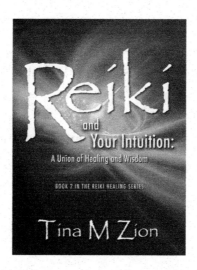

More than just another Reiki book, *Reiki and Your Intuition: A Union of Healing and Wisdom* is a step-by-step process for exploring your intuition, your heart, and your soul as Reiki touches your life, enters your experience, and becomes a part of who you are.

This manual will assist you, as a practitioner or a teacher, in understanding all the strange and sometimes weird and scary intuitive perceptions that Reiki opens you up to. Using a clear and knowledgeable framework presented in this book, prepare to become a better healing vessel as you discover the beautiful union between healing and intuitive wisdom.

Within the covers of this book, you will:

- Find spaces to privately document your heightened awareness.
- Realize what intuition truly is and the keys to being a successful intuitive Reiki practitioner.
- Learn that your intuition is awakened by the Reiki attunements.
- Begin to utilize all the intuitive pathways to assist others and yourself.

- Learn that thoughts and emotions are a vital key to illness, suffering, and wellness.

- Find out why empaths suffer and what to do to help yourself and others.

- Protect yourself in a new way.

- Create a sacred union with intuition and the wisdom of Reiki.

Blank Pages for Your Notes